Chemical

Hypersensitivity

Chemical and Electrical Hypersensitivity

A Sufferer's Memoir

by JERRY EVANS

Foreword by
WILLIAM J. REA, M.D.

McFarland & Company, Inc., Publishers
Jefferson, North Carolina, and London

LIBRARY OF CONGRESS CATALOGUING-IN-PUBLICATION DATA

Evans, Jerry.
    Chemical and electrical hypersensitivity : a sufferer's
memoir / by Jerry Evans ; foreword by William J. Rea, M.D.
        p.   cm.
    Includes bibliographical references and index.

    ISBN 978-0-7864-4770-1
    softcover : 50# alkaline paper ∞

    1. Evans, Jerry—Health.   2. Multiple chemical sensitivity—
Patients—United States—Biography.   I. Title.
RB152.6.E93   2010
362.196'970092—dc22   2010028164
    [B]

British Library cataloguing data are available

Front cover ©2010 Shutterstock

Manufactured in the United States of America

*McFarland & Company, Inc., Publishers
  Box 611, Jefferson, North Carolina 28640
  www.mcfarlandpub.com*

This book is dedicated to all those health-care providers, especially those who had to fight to keep their medical license, who dare buck the trend of drug-fixated symptom treatment that pervades modern Western medicine. It is also dedicated to those healthy people — spouses, family and friends — who do not abandon the sick in their time of greatest need.

And in memory of friends who lost their lives to environmental illness:

Wing L.
Andrew
Linda J.
Eve B.
Kim P.
Selene A.
Monika Q.

If one comes across a person who had been shot by an arrow, one does not spend time wondering about where the arrow came from, or the caste of the individual who shot it, or analyzing what type of wood the shaft is made of, or the manner in which the arrowhead was fashioned. Rather, one should focus on immediately pulling out the arrow.

— Buddha (Shakyamuni), quoted in *The Art of Happiness* by the Dalai Lama and Howard Cutler

A new scientific truth does not triumph by convincing its opponents and making them see the light, but rather because its opponents eventually die and a new generation grows up that is familiar with it.

— Max Planck, German physicist and Nobel Prize winner

I have friends who work in healthcare — I won't mention in which capacities — and when we meet in town we don't greet one another. People at their workplace, the general hospital, are unaware that they are electro-hypersensitive — and they don't dare mention it!

— Testimony at public hearing about electrosensitivity in Sweden, March 8, 2000, from *Black on White: Voices and Witnesses about Electro-hypersensitivity, the Swedish Experience* (Sweden: Mimers Brunn Kunskabsforlaget, 2004)

Acknowledgments

I cannot possibly list all the people who made it possible for me to go on. Many, many people have shown me kindness and understanding, like the clerk in a store who goes the extra mile or the neighbor who picks something up for me in town when I could not go myself. To only mention a few: Dr. William Rea, Dr. Sherry Rogers, Deborah Singleton, Mark Jackson, Don Hules, Karlene Coyan, Ed Blouch, Jim White, John Crawford, Tommie Goodwin, Randy Humber, Jacqueline Colson, Pam Klopfenstein, Connie and Bill Hecht, Russell Friend, Susan Molloy, Bruce McCreary, and especially my parents and my brother. Also a special thanks to the folks who made it a family project to type this book, but who wished to remain anonymous.

The sale of this book benefits the Arasini Foundation of Richardson, Texas.

Table of Contents

Foreword

The author is an engineer who developed electrical sensitivity while doing his line of work. He wrote his odyssey toward health and he has written a classic description of an electrical sensitivity problem in the world today. This problem is growing worldwide and is now only being recognized as a severe problem in some people. Unfortunately, the treatment for those made severely ill by electrical sensitivity is at times very difficult. This treatment involves not only a massive avoidance of electrical generators of any type including cell phones, TV, computers, fluorescent light, power lines, power boxes, etc., but also pesticides and usually many of the toxic chemicals in our environment. In addition, good nutrient programs and a talented energy worker like the one he had (Ms. Debby Singleton) aid in recovery. Also, it helps when the patient is an excellent observer and a person who can innovate recovery. He remodeled his car and home to have less electrical exposure. He had to move to an area with minimal electrical activity. This type of avoidance therapy is extremely difficult as the earth gets smaller and more electrified.

— William J. Rea, M.D., FACS, FAAEM
Founder and President of Environmental
Health Center — Dallas

Preface

Computers fascinated me since before high school, so I became a computer engineer.

About 1996, at the age of 35, I became sick with multiple chemical sensitivity. I was able to continue working while going from doctor to doctor trying to find help — or even just find one willing to discuss a controversial illness.

Eventually I found competent doctors, but by then it was too late. The illness had gotten worse and progressed into electrical hypersensitivity, which meant I could no longer watch TV, use a computer or even stand next to someone using a cell phone.

At the age of 39, I had to check out of regular society and flee to a refugee camp in Texas. Later, I moved to a remote part of the Arizona desert where there are communities of fellow patients. Here we can live in relative peace from the chemical and electrical pollution that makes us sick.

Along the way, I met over a hundred people with the same illnesses, each with their own story. This is my story, and some of theirs too.

Introduction

Imagine getting a flu that doesn't ever quite go away and intensifies when you go into certain stores, buildings, cars and even homes. An illness that is made much worse by everyday things, such as computers and laundry detergent. Then imagine getting it so bad you have to abandon your home.

Meanwhile, the physicians one expects to try to help turn out to be a part of the problem, refusing to take the illness seriously.

Western medicine is based on a mechanistic view of the human body, with a focus on drugs and surgery and little regard for preventing illnesses. Even today, there are doctors who look with suspicion on their colleagues who bring nutrition, acupuncture and other alternative methods into their practice.

Most people who have gone through a serious illness are familiar with the haughty attitude of many doctors. Try to imagine showing up with an illness that is neither understood nor accepted by mainstream medicine; one whose very existence might even question their present world view. An illness that is a threat to large industries, such as those producing chemicals, building products, electronics and telecommunications.

I will admit that if I had not experienced the symptoms of chemical and electrosensitivity myself, it would be difficult for me to accept them as real, but the determined skepticism of the doctors I encountered was also hard to fathom. My view of the world and life itself has been changed in the process of dealing with this illness.

It is my hope that this book can be a comfort and inspiration to those in similar circumstances. Just knowing that others have gone through it before can be a tremendous comfort. Perhaps this book can also be a help in convincing doubting family members and friends.

Although I have typed on computers since 1981, this story was written in pencil and then typed on a manual typewriter. The reason for this cumbersome method will be evident to the reader.

Many people are mentioned in this book. For the sake of privacy, most of their names have been altered. The real names are used for some doctors, while the rest have been designated random letters.

—Arizona, Fall 2010

1

The Road to Dallas

The car was packed the night before, and I only had to load the last few things before leaving. It was a beautiful, sunny fall morning, the first Friday of October 1999. I had packed for a four-week trip — that is what they had told me to expect.

The cooler with my foods and vitamins was quickly loaded, and I closed up the apartment. Soon the skyline of Columbus, Ohio, was fading away as I sped west on Interstate 70.

As I was nearing Indianapolis, it was time to put more gas in my little silver Integra. I hated going to gas stations, but if I was careful, I should do just fine. The whole procedure was well rehearsed by now, developed through trial and lots of pain.

I located a big new gas station along the freeway. It was likely to have the pumps that allow payments by credit card, which were now becoming common. I picked up the respirator from the passenger seat and put it on my face, as I drove off the freeway. I have done it so often, I could do it one-handed now.

The place was not busy. Good. I pulled up at a pump on the edge of the station; it is safer than those in the middle. And yes, it did have a slot for the credit card, so I could get away fast.

In well-rehearsed movements, I pulled out a disposable glove for my right hand, and with a credit card in my left hand, I stepped out of the car. With the left hand, I stuck the credit card in the slot, and pushed the buttons with the gloved right hand. Then I used the right hand to set up the fuel hose, lock the handle and stepped back, waiting for it to fill up.

Nobody seemed to pay any attention to me. I didn't like to be stared at, though most people were really nice about it. I could see it in their eyes: the surprise, the slight startlement, then the averted gazes. The kids would stare in amazement, then ask Mommy. Some parents would hush them up; others would explain that the man over there probably had allergies.

I once had a woman pull up behind me in an SUV. When she saw me, she sat there and stared intently at me until I drove off. Only then did she dare leave her car. I might as well have been a little green man refueling my spaceship.

The tank was full and I put the fuel hose back with my gloved hand. Then I peeled off the glove and threw it in the trash can.

There was an empty open area down the street. I drove there and stopped. I stepped out and opened both doors, before removing my mask. I had a number of times left a gas station and taken off my mask, just to discover there were lingering fuel vapors inside the car. I was so sensitive to gasoline that even a little was enough to trigger a reaction. For hours I would have a migraine-like headache, with the sensation of a nail stuck in my head, and my vision going wobbly on me. Thinking became really hard, as if my mind was inside a drug-induced fog. Sometimes the right side of my face would feel numb too.

The only way to know it is really necessary to do this airing out of the car is the hard way. A single breath of these vapors is often enough to trigger the whole reaction, so I just had to do it every time.

A couple of times I was even able to smell the gasoline fumes from a gas station that was more than two hundred yards away, upwind from me, with nothing in between other than empty farm fields. Perhaps someone had spilled fuel there recently; I don't know. I had no wish to get any closer.

Just driving away from the gas station with the window open, to vent out the fumes, would not work, as the traffic fumes then would bother me. My car was sealed off tightly, with the air intake to the cabin sealed with aluminum tape. Just setting the controls on "recirculation" was not tight enough.

It was only a year ago I had to stop driving with the windows open, which I otherwise preferred to do. Even on the freeway in the open country, I would sometimes on a calm day be bothered by the diesel exhaust by trucks so far ahead I couldn't see them. The first time I noticed that was when I drove home from visiting Dr. Rogers in Syracuse, New York.

I found Dr. Sherry Rogers through her many books. Finally here was a doctor who had a clue about these things, so I went up to visit her clinic in November 1998. That was an experience. Here were other patients with problems being around everyday chemicals. Patients who also would get headaches, blurry vision, the inability to think clearly and other symptoms, if they were in a room with someone wearing perfume, or the carpet on the floor was new. Just going there to meet other people like myself was worth the trip. It was like staying in a foreign country with a different culture, and then suddenly running into someone from your home town.

I told Dr. Rogers that the shots I got from my allergist often would make me dizzy. Sometimes so much that I had to wait an hour before I dared drive home. I had found that I did better if I had eaten right before the injection, but sometimes that wasn't enough. She did a skin test for phenol, the preservative that most allergists use, and it was positive. No wonder.

Then they tested me for various pollen and mold allergies. It took place in a special room with a large stainless steel air cleaner. In the ceiling hung some big ultra violet tubes that would be on all night and kill any mold in the room, all to make sure the patients being tested would not get symptoms from other things than what they were tested for. The testing was much more detailed than at the allergist's. Only one thing was tested at a time, and they wanted to know of any symptoms that developed. The test was repeated with various strengths, so they had an accurate measure of how allergic I was to the various things.

If I got a bump on my arm when they injected me with strength "2," they would do it again with strength "3," which was only a fifth as strong. If I still showed a bump, they would continue with number 4, which was five times more dilute than 3. That is, number 2 is twenty-five times as strong as number 4.

The friendly nurse told me that their patients typically would show mold and pollen allergies around level 4 or 5. But I saw us swiftly move up to 7, 8 and even 9. The highest I scored was 11, on some type of grass. The nurse told me that when men show up there from out of town, we tend to get higher scores as we try to tough it out longer before seeking help.

Of course, I wondered what was the all-time top score. It was an amazing 21! There could not be many molecules left at that dilution.

Then they asked me to write down what I ate every day, and what I ate commonly. I was then skin-tested for that. I didn't know I had food allergies, but the big red welts on my arm spoke their unmistakable language.

Now Dr. Rogers showed me that I was allergic to everything I ate. The only type of food I knew I was allergic to was maple syrup. Almost five years earlier, I once had a nice pancake breakfast and nearly passed out. It took some experimentation to find out it was the maple syrup, but it made sense as I was already allergic to various types of trees. I rarely had pancakes anyway and just never touched the syrup again.

With the revelation that I was highly allergic to beef, chicken, wheat, rice, onions, potatoes, corn, etc., I was instructed to not eat any of it any more. And to take lots of vitamins, as I would be deficient due to the stress my digestive system had been under, constantly having to deal with food I am allergic to.

I did as she told me, but it was hard to completely change my diet. Fortunately, a new health food supermarket had just come to town — Wild Oats. They had many types of food I had never even heard of. Grains like quinoa, millet and teff, meats like ostrich and buffalo, and many kinds of vegetables— grown without pesticides.

Dr. Rogers also instructed me to not eat the same every day, as I would then soon become allergic to that too.

It was a lot of work cooking three meals a day. I could have a bowl of steamed wild rice with fresh squeezed orange juice in the morning, millet with raisins for lunch, and buffalo with celery root and other vegetables for dinner.

I was fortunate that my management had allowed me to work from home three days a week, so it was a lot easier to manage the meals. The days I went in to work, I would bring along wheat-free breads, fruits or dried fruits. My favorite restaurant, the Tandoori Chicken, was very nice to combine meals that would work for me. They were located in a food court with good ventilation, so I did well there most of the time, as long as I avoided the lunch crowd.

After avoiding wheat for nearly two months, I tried to cheat. I had one of their delicious Indian Nan breads. My nose stuffed up, my eyesight got wobbly and when I stood up, my sense of balance was affected. I was amazed; my body had de-adjusted to wheat and showed me what it really thought about it.

The treatment did seem to help on several symptoms. My sinus infections became less severe and I could avoid the usual round of antibiotics. In Dr. Rogers' books, I read about the damage antibiotics do to our digestive system, making food allergies worse, so I was glad to be free of them.

Every winter, I would get a red rash around my mouth, which would go away by spring, all by itself. Each year it became larger, but this past winter, on the new diet, it never showed up.

Another symptom that disappeared were little bumps that now and then would appear around my facial hair. It was easy to pull out the hair, sack and all, and then the bump would go away.

I also started to lose weight. I had slowly been gaining weight over the previous years, probably because I found out that keeping my blood sugar levels high allowed me to tolerate places that otherwise bothered me, so I ate granola bars between meals and sometimes simply had to throw calories at my problems when I needed to perform. Sometimes I counted on the effect, like a time I went to a restaurant with a colleague, and started to feel a little dizzy there, but stayed hoping the food would help, as it did.

Another benefit of this new diet was that I stopped getting deposits on my teeth. For years my dentist had to remove them at each visit, but no more now. I also used to be constantly thirsty and had to keep drinking water.

This was all encouraging. I just hoped it would get to the symptoms that really bothered me, besides the sinuses that seemed to do better. For several years, I would get this "flu" every winter, late in the season. Each year it would linger longer and longer, until spring seemed to take it away. This past spring, it never lifted.

When I visited Dr. Rogers again, ten months later, I had lost forty pounds. Her staff were amazed. But I wasn't really doing better overall. Some of the problems had gone away, but my sensitivity to minute amounts of chemicals had become stronger, and a new type of headache had started. It would come on in the afternoon or evening and last until bedtime and be gone the next day. It was like I had a burning needle in my forehead and right temple.

When I went hiking on Sundays with a friend, the burning pain in the head would not appear, though sometimes I would inexplicably become very tired and had to drag myself back to the car.

Dr. Rogers did some expensive lab work, checking something called enzyme p450, and told me she believed I had Multiple Chemical Sensitivity. That did not come as a surprise. She recommended that I go to see Dr. Rea in Texas, who has the foremost center in the world for treating this condition.

Dr. Rogers had a very nice staff, who had all been there several years. They obviously adored her and told me a few stories. They also told me that they had several patients in Ohio. Maybe not so surprising because in the EPA's Toxic Release Inventory for that year, Ohio took the top spot in one of the categories and was number seven overall.

I had been lucky being accepted as a patient at Dr. Rogers' clinic. It was being scaled back so she could concentrate on her books and lectures, so only six new patients were accepted each month. They chose the patients based on whether they thought they could help, and whether the patient had the right attitude. Patients who expected to receive a magic pill were not accepted.

At the end of my second visit to Syracuse, I was going to drive home in the early afternoon on the third day, but then the last skin test was done with soybeans. I was so allergic to them that the test nearly knocked me out, and I was in no condition to drive home. Instead, I stayed another night in the little apartment on top of Dr. Rogers' private residence next door to the clinic. They rented it out to patients who were too sensitive to stay at a motel or a bed & breakfast they cooperated with. It was a very spartan place with hardwood floors and a tiny kitchen.

Now I found myself on the road to yet another doctor, after seeing three allergists, a surgeon, two chiropractors, an acupuncturist, some pain specialists, etc. But now I finally seemed to be on track and my hopes were very high.

As I drove around Indianapolis on the I-465 beltway, I passed a bill-board with a picture of a sinking ship and the slogan that cigarettes kill more Hoosiers every year than went down with the *Titanic*. The *Titanic* movie was the big box office hit that year.

That was the first time I saw anti-smoking advertising in the Midwest. We'd come a long way there, but it took thirty or forty years from when medical science first sounded the alarm. It would be great if we didn't have to wait so long this time. The tobacco companies were able to delay the reckoning for decades by lobbying politicians and funding "cigarette science." Finally, it was the tide of public opinion and the courts that cut them down. It wasn't the health authorities, beyond some warnings from the Surgeon General.

The same happened with asbestos. The term "asbestosis" was coined by a British physician in 1890, and by 1935, the illness was fully defined and accepted by the medical community. Still, the usage of asbestos kept growing, while the manufacturers paid researchers to cast doubt upon the consensus from 1935.

I wondered how long it would take before everyday products would be made safer, when a new chemical compound was no longer considered safe until proven unsafe by someone else, and it wasn't acceptable that they contain known carcinogens.

I had recently heard on the radio that the tap water in Columbus, Ohio, had repeatedly exceeded the acceptable limits of pesticide content in the last year. There is a lot of farmland upstream from Columbus, with runoff of farm chemicals being carried to the city's water reservoirs by four rivers and major streams. I could be smug knowing that the filter on my kitchen sink would have stopped the pesticides, along with the other stuff that made unfiltered city water taste terrible — until you got used to it. But it is not fair to everybody else. And what is "acceptable levels" anyway? They are based on what doesn't seem to affect lab rats and healthy young men, but what about small children or frail older ladies?

Some of our problems with rising rates of asthma, cancer and other diseases seem to be caused by the release of chemicals by all sorts of products used to build our houses, and make our clothes, entertainment electronics, cars, cosmetics and so much more. Even though the concentrations of these chemicals in the air we breathe inside our houses and offices are low, we breathe it in 24 hours a day, and it can be dozens or more compounds at the same time.

We are a bit like Mickey Mouse in *Fantasia*—unleashing powers we really do not understand or have full control over. Often, we do not use things wisely either. Recently, I saw one of my neighbors go out on their porch and spray insecticide up in the air in all directions, to make a curtain against any bugs. Then they sat down and ate their pizza. Wonder how much of that insecticide landed on their pizza?

Or a co-worker I shared an office with for awhile. She once got irritated by a fly and started shooting it down with a spray can of insecticide, instead of simply swatting it.

Of course, I've done dumb things myself, out of the same blissful ignorance, assuming that if it's available, it must have been checked to be safe by someone. I once traveled to Indonesia and picked up lice somewhere, which I discovered when I landed in Singapore. I had to search for a pharmacy — people there do not consume as many drugs as Americans do. They sold me a bottle of Malathion, which took care of the problem, but had it been today, I would have used Tea Tree oil.

People with Multiple Chemical Sensitivity seem to be like the canary in the coal mine. In the old days, the miners would take a canary with them down into the mines. If the bird fainted, they knew the air was bad and they had to get out before they would be overcome themselves, and possibly die.

Today's canaries are ignored, our message too inconvenient, even threatening to some. Meanwhile, the number of people with asthma is mushrooming, the consumption of pain medication enormous and an unprecedented number of school children have problems paying attention, and I think a lot of these problems are caused by our unhealthy indoor climates and other environmental problems.

2

Accommodation

The Americans with Disabilities Act was created with much fanfare about enabling disabled people to work alongside the able-bodied. I had hardly heard about it and not given any thought of it applying to me. I didn't really think of myself as disabled. The writing on the wall was clear enough, but I still thought of my problems as something temporary that would pass in time, so I would regain the nearly perfect health I had enjoyed most of my life. If I could just find the right fix...

A 1996 trip to New Mexico and Los Angeles had been a wake-up call, but my work life was not really affected yet, except a few minor things, like a co-worker who used perfumes, which gave me a headache.

In the summer of 1997, my work life got suddenly fully involved. I had two offices on campus. One was in the basement of a building where I worked two days a week. The management was slowly restructuring the building and told our group that we would be moved to a new office they were building in a converted storage room. It was next to a large room with the building's air conditioning system, which made it very noisy. The walls were almost vibrating from the powerful motors running next door. Noise has always bothered me; I wondered how anybody would be expected to concentrate on their work in there.

The office was remodeled with a new carpet and new furniture, which smelled strongly. I could not be in there at all. Soon after it was finished, a rain storm flooded the room, which didn't help things either, as a wet carpet is almost a perfect breeding ground for mold.

I thought the new carpet would stop stinking so bad after a few months, so I could move in. I asked the college if I could delay the move a few months. That was granted. My colleague, who spent five days a week in this office, moved and seemed happy enough.

A couple of months went by, and I still didn't do well in there. I started getting comments that it was about time for me to move. I knew I couldn't.

I sought assistance from my local doctor, asking him to write a letter explaining the situation, but he grew very hostile and was not helpful at all.

I got a noise specialist to measure the room. He measured it to be from 53 to 56 decibels; a little high for an office, but not enough that they could help me. Many years later I learned that those instruments ignore the low frequency rumbles, and that only certain people are bothered by them.

Then I went through my own management, the first time ever I had to do that. The way we were set up, I worked very independently with minimal oversight. It was rare I had to ask for things. They came up with the solution that I could simply work from home, using my computer to link up with the university network.

On the rare occasion there was a problem that I could not correct remotely, I could either walk my on-site colleague through it over the phone or drive in and do it myself. The customer would just have to wait the extra time it would take.

I ordered one of the new cable-modems that had just become available that year, so I could have a fast network connection at home, and not have to use a slow modem. It would be installed in early December 1997 and cost a hundred dollars a month to use.

A few days before my official move to work from home, a water pipe burst on the floor above my office and soaked the carpet. I only used the room twice a week, and the carpet had been wet for a couple of days when I discovered it. Then there was a big delay in getting it cleaned up, because the housekeeping department's shop-vac was broken, and nobody had cared to get it repaired. The electrical plug was broken; I got hold of a new one and replaced it in about ten minutes. But the wet carpet had gotten moldy. The housekeeping people said they would take care of it, no problem. The guy poured a gallon of disinfectant over it. I never worked in that office again.

I was much more fortunate with my other customers. I had gotten a new customer, the university library, as my problems being inside many places was surfacing. The computer system they wanted me to manage was located in our main computer room, next to a row of Cray supercomputers. I never had anything to do with the Crays, but since I had access to the room, I often gave tours to colleagues and their families. It was a well-ventilated room with very few people in it, though a couple of the operators wore a lot of fragrances.

The great thing about this new customer was that I never had a need to go to their building, except for our monthly meeting. They cheerfully told me to not even try to enter their offices, and they would be quite happy to come to our meeting room.

This meeting room was located in a building with about seventy people working in cubicles in a large office landscape. I did fine there on weekends and evenings, but during the day I would get tunnel vision within an hour. I had talked with the building manager, who simply told me all regulations were followed, so there couldn't possibly be a problem. The regulations prescribed that 10 percent of the air coming out of the registers must be fresh — not a whole lot. And sometimes delivery trucks would stand idling their diesel engines next to the air intake outside.

I knew most people who worked there, and many complained about headaches, but nothing was ever done. Wonder how much that cost in lost productivity.

The big meeting room in that building had its own separate ventilation system, designed for about forty people being in there, so with only five or six people attending these meetings, I did well there.

My largest customer was a combined central purchasing, warehouse and goods delivering organization, where I had my other campus office. Because of a lack of space, my office was by itself inside a warehouse, while the rest of the organization was in offices next door. My office had no carpeting and the walls were bare concrete blocks, which was great. Some colleagues thought it was a little primitive; I loved it.

I did well there, with some occasional problems. There was a loading area with about a dozen loading docks nearby, and sometimes the big 18-wheelers would stand there idling. The foreman was a nice guy who didn't like air pollution himself. He was good at asking the drivers to turn off their engines.

The dock hands would sometimes leave a pallet loaded with cleaning products near my office, which would give me tremendous headaches, but the foreman was good at limiting this problem too.

That environment gave me some opportunities to check myself. The skepticism I was met with by the doctors couldn't help but make me wonder if I was really somehow imagining it, and I had never heard about other people with this problem. But how to explain that I am fine all day, and then suddenly get sick from a pallet full of laundry detergent or floor wax that was left around the corner, so I could not see it. That happened several times. Or the time someone spray painted a desk in the other end of the big warehouse. It took me a long time to figure out why I was suddenly dizzy with a pounding headache, so when I finally decided to go home, I had breathed so much of it that it took nearly two weeks for me to recover.

Eventually, I became unable to work in that office at all. Just being there, even on weekends with nobody there and the big bay doors open for some fresh air, I would get dizzy and unable to think straight, besides getting tremendous headaches and other symptoms. I first got to that point more than a year after I vacated my office at the other building, and just a few months before my trip to Dallas.

I then worked full-time from my home office, and just came on campus a couple of times during the week — usually at night so I could minimize problems and not be seen wearing my mask. I figured it would just be for a few months, until I had been through the treatment program in Dallas.

Even at off hours, I would sometimes run into "booby traps" at the office. One evening I left the building a minute or two behind one of the office workers, who was working late. A very nice woman, but she really poured on the fragrances. I knew this and never got close to her, but she left a scent-trail behind her in the still air. I should have been smart and put on my mask, but thought it would be o.k. for the minute or so it would take to get to the door. That caused a sinus infection that cost me another round of Amoxicillin antibiotics. At least when I had to wear the mask full-time in the building, I would not run into such problems any more.

My productivity had suffered tremendously in the past year. I did somewhat better working at home, but it wasn't great either. I tried to keep the windows open, as outside air was better than the inside air, despite the work I had done to improve the indoor air quality. But I constantly had to be ready to close the windows again when a diesel truck would show up outside or one of the neighbors would be running their clothes dryer, spewing out a toxic cloud of fragranced detergent and fabric softener. Whoever came up with the slogans about clothes having to smell clean should be shot! Clean has no smell, by definition.

It was like a permanent flu was going on, minus the fever. It would get worse or better, but never go away. I sat at my desk, even though I really felt like staying in bed, but if I didn't try to work, nothing would ever get done. Sometimes I would just vacantly stare at my screen, my mind just being in a haze which we aptly call "brain fog." Anybody who has experienced it, instantly finds the term very descriptive. Someone likened it to trying to think through a brick.

I used to be able to design complicated databases in my head, visualizing how it all fit together, but now I couldn't even frame a letter in my head. Now I had to put down the wording in the word processor, and then use its editing functions to paste it more logically together.

My bosses and colleagues cut me a lot of slack. I felt terrible for needing it. I was used to being the top performer; my work was my life and now I was sinking. A big promotion had been promised, but then it got delayed and finally all talk about it stopped. I can't blame them; I clearly was not up for any challenges. I had looked into moving to a rural university in Ohio, even a research center in the Arizona desert, hoping I would do better in those places. Nothing came of these attempts, which turned out to be for the best. But my hopes were high for this treatment I was going to do in Dallas, so it would just be a rough period before I again could be the performer I had been all along.

3

The Night in Illinois

I had planned to spend the night at Ramsey Lake State Park, about 70 miles east of St. Louis. This far after Labor Day, many parks had closed their campgrounds, but I had checked that this one was open.

I arrived at 3:00 P.M., having saved an hour by passing into the Central Time Zone. It would have been nice to continue a couple of hours more, but it would take that to get to the other side of St. Louis, especially with Friday evening rush hour coming up. And who knows what camping would be like on the other side. I did not have the option of staying in a motel if I couldn't find a usable campground. I had planned the trip with plenty of time to get to Dallas—also so I could rest during the day if the traffic fumes got to me.

The campground office was closed, but a note said that they would be back shortly. After a few minutes, three trucks with some men arrived. Then the ranger returned. I let them all go inside and do their business, while I waited for the place to empty out.

When there was only one visitor inside, I walked in the door, but quickly had to turn around. The place reeked of gasoline. The office was in one end of a small garage building, where they apparently serviced their vehicles.

I waited some more, hoping the ranger would come out on his own, but he stayed inside talking to the last visitor. I took a piece of paper and wrote:

> Sir,
>
> I'm super allergic to fumes from gasoline. I would like to rent a tent-camp site for tonight, much preferably one away from other campers and their campfires. I am on my way to a medical facility in Dallas, which specializes in extreme allergies.

Then I donned my respirator and walked in there. The ranger and the other guy, another park employee, stood right inside the door. Surprise was obvious on their faces. I handed the note to the ranger, while the other

17

employee quickly excused himself. The ranger immediately grasped the situation and quickly issued me a camping permit for their most primitive area. It was a grassy meadow, away from the main campground, and only served by a latrine. No other campers. Perfect. I put up my tent and then cooked dinner on my little camp stove. I hadn't used it for awhile and had to take great care to avoid the fumes from the Coleman fuel. I decided to get rid of it; it is too dangerous to use any longer. Perhaps the little propane stoves would be less offensive.

The dinner consisted of additive-free turkey hotdogs and a boiled rutabaga, with a fresh papaya fruit as dessert.

Another camper showed up after dark and promptly set up a smoky campfire. He apparently used rather wet firewood. I put on my mask and moved my tent as far away as possible. The mask has two charcoal canisters and is great for chemical fumes, but does little for particulates, like smoke from cigarettes and wood fires. It was a calm evening, so there was no place to be upwind from the fire, and the smoke rested like a plume over the clearing. I went for a long walk down the dark, quiet forest road. When I came back, the fire was roaring hot so the smoke went high into the air and wasn't a problem for the remainder of the night.

I was up by first light, and started to pack the car right away. It was a cool 47 degrees, but still no wind. The car was ready to go by the time the sun started to rise a little before 7:00. I wanted to be ready before my neighbor might start a nice morning fire to keep himself warm.

Then I drove over to the main campground and took a shower in a bathhouse. There was nobody else this early in the morning, so I could avoid the fragrances from other people's toiletries, soaps and shampoo. As I was about to finish off by shaving, someone entered who obviously had just finished a cigarette, so I went next door to an unoccupied campsite and plugged in my electric shaver there.

I finally ate my breakfast in the car, and was off. It was easy to drive through St. Louis on an early Saturday morning. After spending half an hour walking around the Gateway Arch and another successful visit to a gas station, I continued further west.

I passed some new buildings going up along the freeway and thought about the strip mall they were building in my back yard. Until this spring it had been a nice green farm field. Then a group of bulldozers showed up and soon a strip mall was sprouting like ugly weeds.

I could watch the work every day, just outside my home office. I had to keep the place closed up when the wind carried the diesel fumes over from the working vehicles. When they poured the concrete flooring and applied some chemicals on top, I had to evacuate for the rest of the day, and first come home around midnight. Even with the windows tightly closed, those strong chemicals seeped right in.

At least they had not started painting the facade yet. Hopefully, that would all be done before my return from Dallas, as that would be really bad to be around for several days.

The flat farmland of Illinois had given way to rolling hills — perhaps the outermost reaches of the Ozarks. It looked a bit like northern Ohio, where a friend had a small farm. His neighbors are Amish. We've sat many a Sunday afternoon on his porch, watching the black buggies run by, with the Amish in their Sunday finest on their way from church service. My friend's wife had jokingly suggested that I join the Amish; they are not fond of modern inventions and fragrances. We had a lot of chuckles imagining me living like they do, with no telephone, no car and no electricity. Hard to imagine such a lifestyle.

Halfway across Missouri, it was time for lunch. The menu items were organic bananas and organic raisins. I had thought I was allergic to bananas, but Dr. Rogers told me that regular bananas are treated with many kinds of chemicals, so I tried organic bananas. I had no problems with them. Then I tried the regular ones again and was rewarded with all sorts of stomach problems, as before. I tried both types one more time; then I was convinced.

Sometimes I have to play detective to find out what the problem is, before I can do something about it. My earliest problem seemed to be my bed. That was years before I'd even heard about dust mites or seen any allergist. I just seemed to get a stomach ache if I lounged in bed in the morning, and then it would bother me for the rest of the day. But if I got up and had breakfast right away, I would have no problem at all. I couldn't explain it, but if that was what it took, that was fine. But it didn't seem to be an issue when I was camping, for some reason.

My girlfriend at the time thought this was really strange, and complained about it. And I couldn't explain why I felt like I did.

I never bothered to tell my doctor. At the time, I wasn't seeing anyone, actually. It was first when my second allergist gave me a catalog with allergy supplies and recommended that I wrap my comforter in an airtight plastic bag, that I suddenly noticed the problem had disappeared. I assume it was dust mites. Now I could frolic in bed on a Sunday morning all I wanted! Later, Dr. Rogers recommended a much better product that is free of plastic. It's called "barrier cloth," which is cotton that has been woven so tightly that even microbes cannot pass through it. It was used in surgical rooms before plastic took over after World War II. It was forgotten for awhile, until someone who was chemically sensitive revived the product. It was certainly much more comfortable than sleeping on plastic, though it cost twice as much.

Life was now more complicated. I had learned to instinctively hold my breath as soon as my nose detected any sort of fragrance or other chemical odor. Then I would have about a minute to walk away from the problem gracefully. I doubt any "offenders" notice anything, when I discreetly walk away.

Sometimes I would have to abandon my place in the checkout line in the supermarket, if a "stinker" decided to line up behind me. The worst was if it happened when my groceries were on the conveyor belt and I couldn't just walk away. Then I either had to endure it, or feign interest in some display rack on the other side of the cashier, or whatever I could think of.

I once wrote to the Big Bear supermarket chain, complaining when a really fragrant cashier gave me a sinus infection. They never replied. That taught me to be more careful checking out the cashier before I committed myself to a checkout line. I was already shopping at odd hours to avoid as many people as possible.

Getting a haircut is another problem. The last few years, I made sure to be the first customer of the day, before the salon got stunk up too much, and I only went to places that didn't do perms. Now that was no longer enough so I found a hairdresser who had her own salon at home, with just one chair. As I continued to be more sensitive, she cut me wearing a mask, and finally she cut me outside on her porch.

The golden colors of the fall leaves started to be replaced by green trees, as I continued further south. More gas was pumped in Joliet, in the western end of Missouri. As I drove out of the gas station, still wearing my mask, an older couple came driving in, passing me closely. They obviously noticed the mask, and in perfect unison turned to look at each other. Then we had passed.

Inside Oklahoma, the landscape turned into range land along the turnpike. By evening I found an RV campground next to a lake. The friendly host told me that the RV'ers never have campfires and rarely use a barbecue. There were a few tent sites along the shore, all empty.

The campground had an ugly restroom with a shower, which was obviously rarely used and in need of some dusting. There was a fragrance dispenser on the wall, so I had to use the respirator inside, despite the open door. I threw the fragrance cartridge out, hoping the place would have time to air out in time for the morning shower.

The next morning, a couple of men were launching a boat before first light. Once they got the outboard started, the oily exhaust drifted over towards my tent. I always kept my trusty respirator within reach for these things.

When another boat trailer arrived, I decided on an early departure. The restroom still stunk strongly of fragrances, and showering while wearing the respirator didn't seem doable, so I did without. Better than having needles stuck in my sinuses for most of the day.

The first light appeared over the lake as I drove off, across the nice masonry dam and back on the highway to the south. The traffic was very light, until I got south of the Texas state line. The highway kept getting wider as I approached Dallas, and it brought me almost to the door of the apartments that are owned by the clinic.

Since many patients come from faraway places, and motels are often not safe enough, the clinic operated eighteen apartments for their patients. Some were two-bedroom units that were shared by two patients, while they also had a few private one-bedroom units.

The complex had around a hundred condominiums in a dense development of two-story buildings enclosing five inner courts. The apartments around one of the courts were almost all owned by the clinic. Years later, the clinic sold these apartments and took over a separate building by a hotel.

The apartments were modified to be safer for people with chemical sensitivities. There was no carpeting, the floors were covered with tiles, and the walls had obviously not been painted for many years. The spartan furniture was basically patio furniture of steel and glass.

There was a television, which was enclosed in a steel box. A fan pulled air through the box and out through a charcoal filter, to absorb the fumes from the plastics, flame retardants, and many other chemicals emitted by electronic equipment.

The tap water stunk heavily of chlorine and tasted like moldy leaves, even worse than what I had back in Ohio. The sink was equipped with a water filter, and there was also a filter on the showerhead, so I would not breathe in the chlorine fumes from the water while showering. There was also a big stainless steel air filter in the living room.

It was wonderful; I did very well in there. A good home for the next few weeks.

4

The Environmental Health Center

Monday morning, I showed up at the Environmental Health Center–Dallas, EHC–D for short. It had satellite offices in Chicago and Halifax, Nova Scotia, and used to have one in Texarkana as well. The clinic is located two blocks from the apartment complex and takes up the whole top floor of one of the buildings on a medical campus across from Presbyterian Hospital. The clinic also has some laboratories in the adjacent building.

The interior was designed to minimize problems caused by building materials. As the clinic expanded over the years, various building materials were used, so it was a showcase of various options for building with low-toxic materials. There was no carpeting anywhere. Instead, the flooring was either ceramic tiles, marble, glazed bricks or a special low-gassing vinyl-like flooring.

The walls in the main hallway were covered with aluminum wallpaper. It had a printed pattern on it, so it was not obvious that the "paper" itself was aluminum. It has since been replaced with ceramic wall tiles.

In the main reception area, the walls were covered with large glass plates, while the walls in the allergy testing rooms and consultation rooms were covered with aluminum porcelainized plates. These porcelain walls were the standard fare in EI-building for awhile, but have since fallen out of vogue. In some of the newer areas, the walls are simply drywall, painted with special paints.

The ceilings were porcelainized plates in the areas where the walls were made of this material, while in other areas, the ceiling was regular ceiling tiles wrapped in aluminum foil.

In an open area was a computer, which was outfitted with a suction hose, that vented the fumes through a charcoal filter, similar to the TV set in my rented apartment.

There is also a store, which is run by an independent foundation. The profit from the store finances research and an annual medical conference held in Dallas. The store sells a lot of books about environmental illness, various clothing and bedding items, high-quality vitamins, chemically free cleaners, detergents, soaps, shampoos, etc., along with water filters, air filters, pesticide-free bug traps, etc. Once a day they get a shipment of fresh bagels from a local bakery, which specializes in making bread from three dozen different types of flour, including quinoa, amaranth, lotus roots, several kinds of beans, etc. The bread is made without yeast and is tasty, but very expensive.

The clinic has a staff of about fifty people, a United Nations of staff members. Dr. Rea's assistant is a cheery doctor from the Philippines. The lab manager is a warm fellow from Puerto Rico with a Ph.D. in molecular biology (I think). The chief of the antigen department, where they produce their own allergy shots, is a woman from Russia. Another doctor is from China. Some of the medical assistants are from India and the Philippines. When I had my initial consultation with Dr. Rea, he had a visiting doctor from Sweden and a medical student from Germany with him.

Dr. Rea is a tireless legend in the circles of environmental illness. A year later, I got to see a list of his life accomplishments, which included being a board-certified heart surgeon, board certified in environmental medicine and a Fellow of eight medical societies. He had held thirteen teaching appointments, including a professorship in England. He has made over a hundred and fifty presentations in sixteen countries and published a handful of books, including a four-volume academic work on MCS, as well as more than a hundred and twenty medical articles. He has received numerous awards that decorate the walls of the clinic.

He has had to fight many political battles with orthodox medicine and is no stranger to controversy, though he rarely expresses it in writing. A fitting quote from an article he co-wrote with Dr. Gerald Ross, M.D.:

> Our understanding of environmentally induced illness is comparable to medical practice 100 years ago, before the germ theory of disease became well-understood.
>
> At that time, people rubbed manure into wounds, and physicians performed pelvic exams after becoming contaminated at autopsies.

Dr. Rea was about 63 years old when I met him, but he seemed much younger. He wanted me to tell the whole story and patiently listened with many questions. Then he asked me to stand up and walk a straight line across the floor, toe to heel. No problem. Then he asked me to repeat it, with my eyes closed. To my surprise, I lost my balance after only two steps. I found out that this little exercise is called the Romberg Test and that virtually every person with MCS fails it.

I was left with his assistant, who told me what would further happen. I soon found out that this clinic is rather lean on staff. The patient is not shuttled around like a mindless child; we are supposed to be active participants and ask questions. A very refreshing approach from the usual medical system that seems to assume that all patients are imbeciles—a warm body that just needs to show up. It was a bit confusing at first, but older patients are a great help in learning the ropes.

The second morning, I arrived on an empty stomach and had blood drawn for a series of tests. They checked my nutritional status, metabolic status, heavy metals and toxic chemicals. There are more than ten thousand chemicals in common use, but since they are expensive to test for, only twenty common problem substances were checked. Of those twenty, I had elevated levels of three of them. On one, I had twenty-nine times the levels in the general population. The levels are really supposed to be zero, but our foods, air and water are now so polluted that there is probably no person on Earth who does not have chemicals in his or her blood. Even animals living in pristine areas, far from human industry, have chemicals and heavy metals in their bodies.

The three chemicals they found that were elevated were commonly used in gasoline, solvents and plastics. No wonder these things bother me so much. And we only checked twenty chemicals—wonder what we missed! I wish we had tested for common chemicals in computers; that would have been interesting.

A lock of my hair was also analyzed, which showed elevated levels of heavy metals as well, confirmed by a blood test. There were metals like cadmium, lead, antimony and strontium that I learned years later are common in computer equipment.

I was spending a lot of money on lab work, but we were learning things. The reports came floating in with all sorts of numbers.

They also checked my autonomic nervous system with a device called an Iriscorder, which measures how fast the iris responds to sudden light flashes.

Another test was called Thermography, where the skin temperature is measured in dozens of points that are associated with various internal organs. I assume these are the same points that acupuncturists use for their needles. Then the skin is briefly chilled, and the same points are measured again. This gives an idea how responsive the individual organs are, and thus their health. The measurements were appropriately done by a doctor from China. The method is, of course, controversial, as is everything that uses the Eastern view of the human body, which orthodox medicine refuses to consider. A fellow patient remarked that the measurement had determined her left ovary to be "unresponsive." It had been surgically removed, but she had not told that to anyone.

My immune response was checked with a rather barbaric instrument that had eight needles on it. Each needle was dipped in a solution containing a weakened organism, such as Tetanus, Diphtheria and Streptococcus. One needle contained saline, as a control. The instrument was pressed hard against my arm, and two days later a nurse read off the response. There were supposed to be seven bumps, showing a healthy immune response. I only got four, with two of them rather small. Some patients get no response at all. A blood test had already shown low levels of white blood cells, so Dr. Rea recommended a rather expensive treatment, called ALF, that was developed by their own researcher. They took another blood sample, from which the white blood cells were extracted. In their lab, they grew more of them, which I got back in a vial four weeks later. They were my own immune system soldiers, and the fiercest of the lot, as only the strongest cells survive the trip through the laboratory. I could now give myself injections from this vial, which temporarily would boost my immune system.

It was potent stuff. A few times I would feel an infection coming on, like a cold. An injection of this stuff, and the invaders were sent packing within fifteen minutes. Amazing! Sometimes when I felt really fatigued, it would give me so much strength I was ready to run laps — once I really did. But these trips to Paradise only lasted about fifteen minutes.

The idea was to prime the immune system to produce more white blood cells on its own, but it didn't happen, and I had to discontinue it after six months. It was simply too expensive to continue.

The level of oxygen in my blood was also checked, and then I was sent on a three-week course of sipping oxygen for two hours every afternoon. The regular oxygen masks are made from very stinky plastic and rubber, so the clinic uses ceramic masks that are hard and not very comfortable. But they didn't make me sick. I did have to boil the Tygon oxygen tube to offgas the plastic, but then it was fine. Some people could never tolerate breathing through the plastic tube and had to use one of steel instead. One woman could not even tolerate the ceramic mask, so one was made for her out of a funnel of stainless steel. She looked hilarious wearing it.

I also tried intravenous infusions of vitamins, minerals and amino acids that boost the detoxification system, so it better can break down the chemicals that are floating around in my blood. The main ingredients were vitamin C, magnesium, Taurine and the amino acid L-Glutathione. The same ingredients Dr. Rogers had instructed me to mix up as powders and

drink when I got sick from exposures. It really helps. When taken intravenously, it bypasses the stomach and works more efficiently. And work it
did. While that drop was stuck in my arm, my mind was as sharp as it rarely
was any more. But the effect only lasted an hour or two after the glass bottle
was empty (plastic IV bags were not used). It was $270 a bottle, so I only
did that a few times. Drinking the ingredients is not as effective, but a lot
cheaper.

I had done a lot of testing for allergy shots at Dr. Rogers' clinic, but I
did some in Dallas as well. There were a lot more available, as they made
them in-house.

Patients could even bring their own substances they were allergic to
and have a custom shot made up. One woman from northern-most Texas
had one made; it was labeled "The North Wind." She explained that she
always felt bad when the wind came down from the north. She didn't know
what the wind carried from that direction, but she rented a machine to
sample the air, from which they produced her special shot.

There are two testing rooms, "A" and "B." Room "A" is where most
people go—the less sensitive. Room "B" is for the most sensitive, who can't
stand to be in "A" because the other people there are not "clean" enough.
Room "A" can hold nearly twenty people, while "B" is a little smaller with
about a dozen chairs.

Even though people are instructed to arrive without any scented products, many of the less sensitive do anyway. Most people do not know that
almost all personal care products sold in a supermarket contain fragrances,
even those marked "unscented." They still contain a "masking fragrance,"
as the products would otherwise be unsellable, as the stench of the chemicals
would make it unpleasant for anyone to smell. The fragrances people use
on a normal day will hang in the clothes even after multiple washings.

When we test for shots, it is imperative not to get the results affected
by other things, as monitoring the symptoms is a part of the test. Some
patients do not even generate the tell-tale bumps that an orthodox allergist
would consider the only acceptable sign of an allergic reaction. The immune
system is simply not up for even that much. Others get symptoms from
lower doses than what creates a bump. I do that myself.

For the really severe, who can afford it, there is a special glass-enclosed
room next to "B," called "the box." It looks like a big aquarium.

Each of the two testing rooms has one or two "testers" on duty. They
test for only one thing at a time, by injecting a small amount under the skin
on the arm. After ten minutes, the injection area is inspected for swelling,
and the patient is asked for any symptoms.

If there is a swelling or a symptom, a new injection is made, but diluted five times. This is repeated until there is no effect from the injection. That is called the endpoint, and is the strength used in the vials we get, so the shots are tailored to the individual. A far cry from the one-size-fits-all allergy treatment I'd been given for 2½ years. These vials are also completely free of any preservatives, so they must be stored frozen.

It was often an interesting crowd in "B," with lots of laughs. The gaiety could quickly change, as people reacted to their next injection and became very quiet. Sometimes the reactions could be severe. A couple of times, people simply passed out. A German woman suddenly started crying uncontrollably, until an assistant came with an oxygen mask to help her out. But mostly it was just itchy eyes, runny noses and various kinds of pain and discomfort.

I tried to test for some of the common chemicals that I was exposed to, such as traffic fumes, ink and smoke from fireplaces. These did not produce skin reactions, so I had to go by the symptoms alone. They were severe. After two or three attempts, I was so messed up I could not tell any difference from further shots and had to call it a day. I spent three days in a row, trying to find an endpoint for ink. I was determined to find a treatment for this important substance that is used in books, newspapers, photocopies, magazines and more. But I had to give up. In the end, I was only able to get shots for a couple of chemicals, and they turned out not to help me anyway. These chemical shots rarely help, but for some patients they do, so it was worth trying.

It was interesting to show up at the clinic every day and see what kind of people would be there. They came from all over the country, as well as foreign nations. Some people came once a year for checkups and could tell stories of earlier times and who had been there, including two Hollywood stars and even a member of the very highest circles of England.

The patients at the clinic were basically all white and middle class, almost none were black, Hispanic, Native American or working class. People who come here have found the place on their own and had the money to pay for it.

One afternoon I was sitting and breathing oxygen in one of the small rooms next to the row of examination rooms. A very fragranced woman walked down the hallway with her little son. Her vapor trail drifted in to our little group and made us all sick, despite hurrying to shut the door. Emotions ran high; we were all indignant. How could the clinic personnel allow such a stinker to walk in here, one of the very few places we should be allowed to be free of this menace!

When Dr. Rea walked out from the examination room again, the anger in our little room next door was still rolling. He heard it and came in. He calmly told us that the patient was not the woman, but her little child. If the woman had been turned away by the staff, it was unlikely that she would have returned, and her son would have been doomed to a life of drugs and misery because of the woman's toxic lifestyle. Then he just left the room, with all of us very quiet for a bit. Then we quickly agreed that a few hours of pain on our part was worth it for saving the child.

5

From Doctor to Doctor

I was extremely healthy as a child and up through college. My brother got all the childhood diseases we are supposed to get, while some of them didn't affect me. My only problem was that I easily got motion sickness in cars, boats and airplanes.

My work with computers gave me wrist problems after some years out of college. My wrists became so inflamed it was interfering with my work. I went to doctors who prescribed massive doses of Ibuprofen and gave me steroid injections. Much later did I learn that all that Ibuprofen was a possible factor in the severe food allergies I later developed, through what is called Leaky Gut Syndrome.

In retrospect, I probably did have some food allergies as far back as college, but it didn't bother me much and was never diagnosed.

The drugs the doctors gave me for my wrists didn't work for long. Then they sent me for some expensive physical therapy, which was worthless. The doctors never suggested looking at my work setup; I had to think of that myself. Ergonomic keyboards were expensive and not easy to find in those days. I bought one for $400 that was made in Germany. At work I got a better setup, and someone told me about a special glove he had read about. It was made for people who do needlework, which is also hard on the hands, and it helped greatly.

This was my first experience with the way much of modern medicine tries to solve difficult problems. It is like noticing a warning light on the car's dashboard when driving down the freeway. The prudent response is to take the car to a mechanic immediately and correct the problem. The standard medical method is to take a roll of masking tape (in the form of a pill) and cover up the offensive warning light, then tell the car owner to keep going. Perhaps suggesting going a little slower, but go on anyway. If something major happens down the road, they will happily do surgery to remove the burned-out part. The truth is that most medicine is only treatment of the symptom. Its practitioners do not attempt to correct the problem that caused it in the first place. Of course, patients are at fault here too. It is much easier to take a pill for high blood pressure, rather than looking at diet, perhaps losing some weight, start exercising and lower the stress levels. A pill is much more enticing, and the medical system is quite happy to dole them out so they can get on with the next patient.

I was guilty of this way of thinking myself. My first warnings were perhaps some stomach problems that went away again, followed by a burst appendix and then a kidney stone, but I wasn't really interested in that. Just glad the fellows in the white lab coats would take care of it, so I could continue with what interested me.

It was when I passed thirty that allergies first became an issue I took notice of. I wasn't used to going to doctors. They gave me a prescription, and the problem went away. When it stopped working, I got another prescription. I wasn't really concerned; the doctors were busy, so I didn't ask much. The doctors never told me about allergies or volunteered much else.

After a year or two, it wasn't working any longer. A friend talked me into visiting her allergist. He was very nice and filled my back with a lot of little pricks with various kinds of pollen extracts. There was no doubt: I had allergies to many things. He gave me a prescription to try, and another when that didn't work. Meanwhile, my allergies got worse, so he started me on weekly allergy shots. I faithfully did them for 2½ years. Still, I kept getting worse. Slowly, but surely. When I asked about the lack of progress, I was told to be patient. Well, he must know, he is the doctor.

One Saturday morning in the spring of 1995, I did my usual weekly stroll over to a nearby supermarket to buy a newspaper. It was about a mile over there. When I arrived, I was so mentally confused that I hardly knew which way was up or down and could barely stay on my feet. I did have enough sense to call my girlfriend on the phone. She was out in the yard, but picked up the message on her answering machine soon after. She later played it for me. I sounded like an incoherent drunk and didn't really tell her anything beyond that I wasn't doing well. She, of course, knew that I usually walked to the supermarket and came to pick me up, finding me staring vacantly at the wall next to the payphone. At home, with an air filter going, I quickly recovered.

The allergist told me that Ohio was experiencing an unusually high concentration of tree pollen that spring, so better stay inside until it calms down again. During this period, I would get a headache whenever I stayed outside for more than fifteen minutes.

A week or two later, I drove to the supermarket. I felt the same dizziness coming on again as I walked in the parking lot. There was a walk-in clinic across the street, so I staggered over there. I hadn't been to any other doctor than the allergist for awhile, and I was now seen by a physician I had never met before. I was feeling very crummy, nauseated and unsteady, but he just said I was fine, as if it was stupid of me to come here. When I asked him if it could be the allergies, he categorically stated that everybody who walked in there thought they had allergies, it was just a fad. I certainly did not have allergies. When I told him that my allergist had another opinion, he huffed some comments and promptly left the room.

I used to go to a monthly meeting with other computer people, who did the same kind of work that I did. We met in a building that I otherwise never went into. Most times, I left the meeting with a headache, but now I was used to those from my allergies. Before my allergies became a problem, it was very rare for me to have a headache or any other pains.

During one meeting, my headache got worse than normal, and I started to feel really nauseated. I decided I needed to get some fresh air and left before the meeting was over. Once I stood up, I felt worse and my sense of balance seemed off. I staggered down the hallway, couldn't keep upright and slumped into a chair in an empty office. I was so nauseated I felt like I would throw up if I did any movement of my head. I could see our director in a nearby office. With great care not to move my head much, I called him for help. He took one look at me and wanted to call 911, but I declined. Two colleagues drove me home, and I felt awful for three days; then I was fine again. Some people told me that this building did not have good ventilation. I did not attend any more meetings there.

I did tell the story to a doctor in our walk-in clinic, a young woman who could not have been long out of medical school. She just shrugged it off, saying I probably had not drunk enough water that day. She was not interested. I would have respected her more if she had admitted that she didn't know, instead of giving such a dumb answer.

I have found that only truly competent professionals have enough integrity to admit that there are things they do not know. That is a yardstick I use to judge both myself, my colleagues and physicians. Regrettably, only a few doctors have measured up. Dr. Rogers is one. Another is an eye doctor I went to when I started having disturbances of my eyesight, before I figured out it was caused by exposures to chemical fumes. He readily admitted he had no explanation for what made my eyes blurry and made light surfaces, such as the wall of his office, seemingly come alive. He even told me that he had seen another patient with the same symptoms. The third truly professional doctor is Dr. Rea, though it took many, many questions before there was something this remarkable man could not answer. I have much later met a couple more.

In the fall of 1995, I spent some time in Australia and Southeast Asia. The cities of Bangkok and Kuala Lumpur were highly polluted, with the air having a distinct bluish color from the exhaust fumes of the many two-cycle engines. I felt sick around rush hour in the center of the city and had to buy a facemask from a street vendor. The traffic police in Bangkok wore masks during rush hour themselves. I am really glad I got to do all this travel, before my illness made it impossible.

I used to go backpacking a few times each year. During one backpacking trip to a wilderness area in West Virginia, we started to get attacked by mosquitoes when we set up camp for the night. I brought out a bottle of bug repellant and started applying it to my skin. That gave me a big headache, so I had to go without.

I was getting warnings, but didn't heed them. And the doctors didn't care.

By the summer of 1996, my allergies were a major problem. I had become extremely sensitive to grass, so I would get dizzy when passing someone mowing their lawn. The fragrances people wore were now also bothering me. Though I've never liked them, they were now a real problem.

I went on vacation to Albuquerque, New Mexico, thinking that perhaps I could move there, that a desert city was better. I didn't do any better in the city itself, but noticed that my sinuses would clear up if I went to the western city limits, where the wind came in from the open desert.

I flew in late on a hot Friday evening and picked up my rental car in the airport. I was surprised how much it smelled of "new car." It was terrible; I could hardly breathe in it. I opened the windows and drove out of the parking ramp. It was past 11:00 P.M., and I was really tired from the long flight. My motel was just down the street. I would deal with it tomorrow. Tomorrow it would be just fine.

The motel had freshly installed carpeting in my room. I thought it smelled very strongly, and unpleasantly. It was so late, I was so tired, and I didn't know what it all meant. Surely, it would be just fine in the morning. I popped a couple of pills I was on at the time — Seldane and a decongestant — and went to bed. (Seldane has since been found to be too dangerous and taken off the market.)

The next morning I couldn't walk a straight line out to my car. After being outside for awhile, it cleared and I could drive. The new-car smell was still strong and really bothered me, even with all the windows open. Only on the freeway was there enough ventilation for the car to be fine.

I drove back to the airport and told the story to the friendly people at the Budget car-rental counter. They didn't think my problem was strange and cheerfully handed me a stack of keys and offered me to pick any car that would work for me. I had to try a few, before one didn't seem to bother me. When I returned to the counter, they told me I had chosen their oldest car; it was due to be phased out. I did very well in that car for the week that I drove around New Mexico. I slept every night in my trusty old tent and had a great vacation, though I noticed the areas I felt the best in were devoid of trees and human activities.

From Albuquerque, I flew on to Los Angeles, to attend a computer conference. The carpet in my hotel room there was also a problem. The staff told me it was about 18 months old and gave me another room where the carpet was three years old. It also had a balcony, so I could keep the door open at night. That worked, though the polluted air outside would bother me during the day when I walked to the conference center.

When I got home to Ohio, I discussed these events with my allergist. He didn't have much to say about it and was not very interested. It was then I realized that I had been very wrong, relying on the medical system. Even though it is set up so we are encouraged to passively just do what the doctors tell us, that is not the way to get anywhere. I had to take charge of my own health. I had to learn what this is all about.

I contacted the American Academy of Asthma and Allergy to get more information, including how to find a more competent doctor. I had now been to two allergists and received shots for 2½ years, and still was steadily losing ground.

The problem took on more urgency as more things started to bother me. Now I would get dizzy and have tunnel vision if I spent more than an hour in my boss's office.

I found an allergist with lots of credentials. I went to him and was initially impressed. He took his time and listened to my story. Then he did a completely new set of allergy tests. He went through his cabinets and gave me a whole bag full of samples of all kinds of allergy drugs to try. I went home and tried them. Nothing was helpful.

The new shots were made up and given to me once a week. The allergy clinic was only open during the day, so I would have to take off at least an hour every week to do the shots. Instead, I got the walk-in clinic to administer them to me on my way home from work. They made me dizzy, sometimes so much that I had to wait an hour before I felt comfortable driving. They kept lowering the dose. One of their nurses seemed to blame me for not doing well on the shot, when she gave it to me, and she highly disapproved when I asked them to lower the dosage.

Finally, the dose was as small as they would make it, and I was pretty much told to take it like a man or don't take it. I was determined to get better, so I let them do it and didn't say anything about the effects, even when asked.

A sympathetic nurse later told me that they had once given me a saline injection to see how I did. I did fine, so it wasn't some sort of psychological problem. She was much friendlier than the other nurse, so I made sure to come on the days she was there. She suggested I try to eat something before I got there, and that was excellent advice.

I started getting headaches when I was sitting in their waiting room, even if I sat all by myself. I spent a lot of time there. It always seemed to take about an hour, regardless whether the waiting room was empty or full. It is first when we get sick we realize why the word "patient" has two meanings. Eventually, I noticed that I did fine on Mondays, but not the other days. I told the observation to the staff, and asked if they knew of any difference between Monday and the rest of the week. The response was as if I had asked an obscene question.

Finally, the sympathetic nurse came up with a likely explanation. They had a cleaning crew coming in every morning, except Monday, as the place was closed on Sundays. Perhaps the cleaning agents were a problem for me. I asked my doctor about it, but he didn't want to discuss it. Nor did he want to talk about my increasing problems with perfumes, which by now seemed to give me sinus infections that often required antibiotics.

The next spring was the best in several years. The shots did seem to help. When I told the allergist, he seemed surprised.

That summer, I went to another computer conference, this time in Chicago. I was one of the speakers and had to submit a paper in advance. I was working on it late in the winter, which always is the worst time of the year for me. This year I felt tired for months and had a hard time gathering my thoughts. The shots had not done anything to help that, only the pollen allergies. It was a real chore to finish the paper, but I did. I had published a dozen articles in computer magazines over the previous years but had to stop, as I no longer had the mental energy to do it.

During the conference, I was to stay four nights at a fancy hotel nearby. I remembered the unpleasant experiences I had had with the hotels in Los Angeles and Albuquerque the previous summer, so I called up the hotel in advance and explained the problem. They told me that they would give me a room with an operable window and not let anybody use the room the night before, unless they got full. That way the cleaning agents would have had time to dissipate, and there would not be anything left over from the previous guest. No problem.

When I got there, the room gave me a headache within ten minutes, and the window was bolted shut. I could not open it. The front desk said they would send up a serviceman to increase the airflow into the room. He got there quickly and was a nice fellow who understood the problem. The two portable air cleaners I had brought with me also helped his understanding that this was a real problem.

He removed a wall panel and showed me how the room air was pulled in through one register, through a radiator for heating and cooling, and then back into the room. The only fresh air that ever entered the room was under the door to the hallway, and that was only when the bathroom exhaust fan was running. The bathroom fan was controlled by a timer and only ran a couple of hours each day. Basically, there was no fresh air coming into the room.

It really surprised me that such a fancy hotel had no fresh air coming into their rooms. They had a huge glass-covered atrium, concierge service and all sorts of other services, but no fresh air.

The friendly serviceman told me he would get permission to open the window, which could only be opened with a special key. He called up his director, got permission, and then opened the window. I did fine there the whole four nights, but it was such a hassle.

The first day of the conference, we could choose among a number of all-day lectures and classes. I had chosen a hands-on class about the then-new computer language called Java. The class was held in a room with about 50 PCs, so we could play with the language during the class. All the PCs were brand new. When I had been there a couple of hours, I started to fade. The subject interested me, but I seemed to have a hard time grasping some of the details and concentrate on what was said.

I felt better after lunch, but it got worse in the afternoon. I nearly fell asleep and finally left the room early. Much later did I realize that the problem was probably the fumes from all the new computers in the room. When electronics get warm, they offgas all sorts of chemical fumes, such as plasticizers and flame retardants.

In the fall I traveled to visit an old friend and celebrate Thanksgiving together with him and his wife. He was one of only two people whom I had confided in about my mounting problems, but he wasn't very understanding.

I did fine in their older ranch house, but got concerned when they told me that the Thanksgiving dinner itself would be at her sister's house. He told me not to worry, the place was fine. They would put their pets upstairs so they would not bother me, as I was also allergic to cats.

The sister's house did not work well for me, but we sat down to eat soon after we arrived. I knew food usually made me feel better in places that otherwise would not work for me, and I made it through dinner fine. A couple of hours after the meal, I started to get dizzy again and went for a walk. When I got back, we were ready to go back to my friend's house. On the way back, they told me that the house I had just been in was painted a week earlier. They figured that if I didn't know, it wouldn't bother me.

The next day we put up their Christmas tree, which was made of plastic. We got it all nicely decorated with glass bulbs and electric lights, and that went well. Then we turned on the electrical lights. Soon after that, I got a tremendous headache. We figured out it was the heat from the lights that warmed up the plastic, which made it offgas enough plastic fumes and flame retardants to affect me. It was turned off again, and I was fine for the remainder of the visit.

The university had a special pain clinic. Since my doctor did not seem to be interested in my problems, I went to see them. I met with two of their doctors, but that was fruitless. They must have thought I was stressed out, since they gave me instructions in how to relax, using visualization. That didn't help anything, but it was a nice tutorial and I did use it a few times during stressful periods.

Then I was referred to a specialist, who would take a look at my sinuses. He was in deep conversation with a colleague during the brief time we met. I might as well not have been there. He just looked in my mouth and my nose and then tried to choke me a few times with a swab, before they walked out again. Another complete waste of time. At least my health plan covered the full fee; otherwise, I would have complained.

I now had to get really involved, I had to figure out what the problem was. Apparently, even doctors with high credentials were clueless. I started looking around for medical information. This was the early days of the Internet and there was not much information there, outside the computer field, and the occasional private home page with a picture of some nerd's cat or girlfriend. But I looked around and eventually came across the term Multiple Chemical Sensitivity (MCS). It was in a document about something else. No further description or any references, but it sounded promising. I could not find anything else about it on the net. Perhaps there was, but search engines were very primitive in those days.

I had run across a catalog from a company in New England called Non-Toxic Living (it has since closed) which sold an assortment of paints and other building products that claimed to be healthier. I called them up and asked if they knew what MCS was. The woman told me that they had a book about it. She suggested I buy it and make up my own mind. It was $20, a bit much for a book I knew nothing about, but I ordered it. It was *Living Well in a Toxic World* by Lynn Lawson.

I read the introduction and lost interest. It seemed quite far fetched, that was not me. But now I'd spent twenty bucks on that book, so I decided to read the first couple of chapters anyway. Then I gobbled up the whole book. It described my problems precisely. Now I had something to go by for more information.

I very nearly repeated the mistake I had once made with another book on the subject, called *An Alternative Approach to Allergies* by Theron Randolph, M.D. After reading the introduction, I shelved the book, and first read it years later, when it turned out to be the best introduction to MCS and allergies I have ever read. It is written by the same doctor who discovered MCS back in the 1950s, who was driven out of his academic research position by colleagues who ridiculed and blocked his work. The field of medicine can be especially nasty towards those who dare go against the prevalent orthodoxy. History is full of examples.

At the time, I was seeing some alternative health practitioners, who treated me with acupuncture and various other things. It didn't help my MCS problems, but it did convince me that there was something to acupuncture and homeopathy, especially after I was cured of a week-long bout of stomach flu in less than two hours, just by taking a couple of drops under my tongue.

When I gave up on these attempts, I was ready to try out-of-town doctors. Once I had discovered MCS, I was able to find books about the topic and soon found a book by a doctor in Syracuse, New York. A few months later, I traveled to her clinic.

Dr. Sherry Rogers required her out-of-town patients to have a local physician to cooperate with for blood work and administering her phenol-free allergy shots. Naive as I was in the ways of physicians, I just asked the last local doctor I had seen. She looked like I had poked her with a hot iron.

I once saw pictures of a whole class of medical students at the Ohio State University. They were all seated in wheelchairs, which they had to spend a whole day in, so they could learn something about the patient's perspective. Too bad that tradition since has been forgotten. Today's physician needs to learn compassion.

But my immediate problem now was to find a doctor who would be my local support for drawing blood and administering shots. I had the kit for the blood work, which contained everything needed, including a green biohazard bag for shipping overnight to the lab in North Carolina. But it was difficult to get anybody to draw the blood. I asked the walk-in clinics. They would not do it for a doctor that was not associated with them. Finally, I found a place in the system that would do it, but unofficially. No paperwork, cash payment, it never happened. It was good to see that there were still people who cared.

Then there was the problem with the shots. I didn't know how to do them myself, and Dr. Rogers wouldn't authorize me to do it anyway. A spouse would be fine, but not myself. Also here the walk-in places refused. They were soon to be remodeled anyway and thus would be inaccessible to me.

I found a little clinic that served a low-income neighborhood. One of the physicians there was willing to do it, if the first shot was done in his presence. That worked, though the clientele and the staff were all highly fragranced. I usually had to wait 45 minutes before they called me in, so I had to sit with a respirator on for that long. After going there twice a week for two months, I would get dizzy even when I wore the mask. It is only 90 percent effective. I then had to sit out in the lobby of the building. When I left the building, I had to change my shirt as it reeked of cheap perfume. I would instantly get sick if I left it on, even outside.

I complained about the staff using so much perfume and was told that it was the policy of the place that the staff should not wear perfume. But it was obviously not enforced. One supervisor I talked to asked me to play "fragrance police" and drag any offenders into her office, but that was ridiculous. The friendly physician who was helping me with the shots could just agree that it was undoable to get them to stop.

I would just have to find a solution to that problem once I got back from Dallas. I was optimistic that things would finally turn around, building on the work Dr. Rogers had already done. Here were doctors who were competent and clearly cared about what they did. Just too bad I had to leave the state to find such rare specimens.

6

Sauna

Dr. Rea didn't wait the three weeks it took to get all the lab results back to send me to detox treatment. He has seen thousands of patients and could tell I needed it. I went to the sauna area on the third day, after the initial blood tests were taken, so we could compare with later tests.

The detox procedure was originally developed by a doctor for helping drug addicts getting through withdrawal. Environmental doctors have now used a version of it for decades to pull stored chemicals out of our bodies. The basic problem is that our detoxification system is not able to keep up with the onslaughts of chemicals that enter our bodies through what we eat, drink, breathe, and put on our skin. Healthy people can usually break down the chemicals through a complicated multi-step process and then excrete them. In people who have MCS, one of the stages in this process does not work well, so it cannot keep up. Instead, our bodies store the chemicals it cannot get rid of, hoping to work on them later. But, there is never a "later," as there are few places in the modern world that are free from pollution. So the chemicals keep building up in our fatty tissues and organs, such as the brain, liver, and kidneys, which may get damaged. Most EI's have problems with short-term memory and the autonomic nervous system, which is why we usually can't walk a straight line blindfolded.

When I got to the sauna area, the attendant first weighed me and took my blood pressure. Then I was issued a set of supplements to help my body handle the toxins that were to be released by the heat of the sauna. It was chiefly high doses of Niacin and Vitamin C.

I had to experiment with how much Niacin to take. If I took too much, the skin would burn for about ten minutes, as if I had been in the sun too long.

Then I signed up for a time slot in the sauna and jumped on an exercise bike. Sometimes I would also use a rowing machine or a treadmill. There was also a stair-climber and a trampoline. The trampoline was rarely used, and mostly by people who did not have the strength to do any other kind of exercise.

The exercise is an important part of the detox procedure, as the muscles help the process along as well. I like to hike, but was not used to this kind of exercise, so I only did ten minutes at first.

After the exercise, I went to the sauna. I started out with a cautious five minutes and quickly ramped it up. After two weeks, I was doing 45 minutes in there, but then the weekly blood test showed my liver was being stressed. I decreased the time to 25 minutes, and the liver was again happy.

After the sauna, we had five minutes to take a quick shower to rinse off the sweat. We were instructed to go directly from the sauna to the shower, so we did not have a chance to cool down and reabsorb some of the toxins that had come out in the sweat. Most people don't know that we absorb things through the skin into the blood stream, but we do. That feature is used by the nicotine patches, for instance, so it's as important to avoid using chemical creams just as it is to avoid chemical foods.

Well refreshed by the shower, I had my blood pressure checked again. The attendant handed me a little cup of salts that I drank to counteract the acidity of my body from the sauna treatment. Then I got more supplements and was offered some vegetable oil as well. The supplements helped my body break down the toxic chemicals that have been brought out into the blood by the sauna treatment and are basically the same "detox cocktail" that I had been using for a year, including more Vitamin C, Taurine and L-Glutathione.

The oil is to build new cells, as the oil we get from processed foods is altered and does not work so well. In my case, I also drank it to stabilize my weight that had dropped 45 pounds over the last year. I was liking my new slimmer self, but I was getting to be a little too thin now.

The final part of the treatment was a ten-minute lymphatic massage. The lymph system is gently helped to excrete the toxins as well.

The whole treatment took me about an hour in the start, and two in the end. On some days, I could do one in the morning and another in the afternoon.

For the past several years, I'd had night sweats of nearly biblical proportions, with my body desperately trying to get rid of toxins. After weeks of sauna treatment, they have never happened again. I was getting cleaned out.

One woman from a large city on the East Coast scared me one day, when she went into seizures. I had never seen that before. She had been poisoned by pesticides, like so many others. Another woman, from a Midwest farm state, had so much pesticide in her that few people could share a sauna with her. She stunk of the stuff even when not inside the sauna.

There was a great sense of camaraderie among the patients, especially when sitting in the sauna — it was the social event of the day. We all told our stories to each other — how we ended up here. It is a good thing to be validated after so many of us have been ignored or even ridiculed by doctors, family, friends, and bosses. I have definitely been much luckier with that than most.

After awhile, the stories become a blur. There are so many similarities. Eventually, it does get tiresome to listen to yet another sad story of pain and what people do to each other, though it is therapeutic to tell the story to people who understand. The clinic had a therapist, and she seemed busy enough.

Some inside humor developed, such as the story about the person who thought that the rotation diet means going to McDonald's on Monday, Burger King on Tuesday, Wendy's on Wednesday and Taco Bell on Thursday. Of course, junk food is a no-no, and what is rotated are the basic food stuffs, such as wheat and beef.

People from other countries told about how it is to live with MCS there. A woman from China told us that she cannot discuss her illness with anyone there. It is a macho culture where the sick are not supposed to show they are sick in any way. Take it like a man, ma'am. She got sick when her office was remodeled with new carpeting.

The sauna treatment can sometimes make a person more sensitive, just as the testing for various chemicals can. The heat of the sauna induces the body to bring out toxins from its stores and release them to the blood stream for transport to the sweat glands and other methods of removal. The amount of toxins in the blood is thus higher during the sauna treatment than it otherwise would be. In his book *Optimum Environments for Optimum Health and Creativity*, Dr. Rea shows on graphs how the toxins go up in the blood during the treatment, then slowly go down again over several weeks.

The increased body load made me more reactive to chemicals, which was quite scary. Suddenly, the polluted air in Dallas was unbreathable to me. It was like I was in a smoky room, just being outside. I could taste the bad air in my mouth; it tickled my lungs, made me dizzy. I had to wear a mask outside, except on weekends when I did fine outside most of the time.

Of course, Dallas is rated one of the most polluted cities in North America, according to EPA data. That year Houston was ranked number one, surpassing Los Angeles, where pollution controls are being taken seriously. Libertarian Texas is famous for their lax environmental oversights, and the Texans love oversize vehicles.

I'd been having problems with printed materials for awhile, especially newspapers, but I could read books if I was a little careful. Now I could not even read a book any more, along with magazines and photocopies.

We got freshly washed linen in our rooms every week. It was washed in "Granny's," a less toxic detergent that many of us used. I had had no problems with it before, but now I couldn't be in the same room as the bedding and had to wash the sheets in baking soda myself.

The towels they issued us in the sauna were also washed in Granny's, so I had to bring my own. It became so bad that I could not share a sauna with other people, who would bring their towels with them. I had to sign up for using the solitary sauna, which I shared a couple of times with other people in the same predicament.

Since I got there, I had had to stay clear of the crowd from testing room "A," many of whom used products that were fragranced. Some were even so bad that they created a vapor-trail of the stuff when they walked down the hallway. I got "hit" very hard by that, when I unwittingly walked into such a booby trap.

Now I even had problems with some of the people in the "B" room! I had to use a mask even there; otherwise, I could not tell whether my symptoms were generated by the injection or something brought in by another patient.

My sense of smell was super-super-charged. It was amazing what I could pick up. Wonder if I could get a job sniffing bags at the airport? Of course, I would not last five minutes in such a place. Fortunately, some of these problems went away a month after I stopped the sauna treatment.

One woman stank terribly of laundry products to me. She told me she had switched to safe products three months earlier; the clothes had been washed many times since. Fabric softeners are designed to be "sticky," but still...

Newcomers were usually a problem, as it is really hard to clean up without someone else to "sniff one out." A new patient came to the sauna smelling like a laundromat. Some people fled the room. I talked with him. He professed his innocence: "I'm clean, man." He might as well have held up a red tee shirt and tried to convince me it was blue. He said they had been washing with baking soda for a long time—it could not be. When I pressed him for details, he did say that he had seen his wife throw "something" into the dryer with the clothes. Aha, dryer sheets! He apparently stopped that practice, but he never got clean enough that I could be near him. Once I could smell him two rooms away, at least it seemed to be him. He even claimed to have bought all new cotton clothing, but they were staying in a hotel and washing in a laundromat, so some must have rubbed off on his clothes from other people's use of the dryers. I simply stayed clear of him and put on my respirator whenever he got near me. My sinuses would be very painful the rest of the day if I got "hit" by that stuff. Apparently, it rattled his cage a lot, judging from his incessant "It's not me, I'm clean, man." Needless to say, I was glad when he left after staying for a couple of weeks.

Another woman also smelled like fabric softener. When I mentioned it, she was surprised and told me that she had never used it, but she would think about it. The next day, she walked up to me, stuck her hair up in my face and asked me to sniff her out. A behavior that would seem odd to outsiders, but is perfectly acceptable here. There was no hint of fabric softener on her. She told me that she was from out of town and stayed at a friend's house. Her friend did use fabric softener on her towels, and from there it got on her when she used the towels. Now she used her own towels and was glad to be free of the unnecessary body burden.

We get so used to our own smells that we don't even notice them any more.

7

Dallas Community

It did not take long for me to set up a comfortable "home away from home" in the little spartan apartment. It was nice to have so many neighbors with the same focus, and they quickly familiarized me with the area, especially where to get organic food. Within five miles, there were no less than three Whole Foods markets, each the size of a regular supermarket, but only selling foods that are safer than the regular fare, and also with an emphasis on ethical food sources.

The shopping was much better than in Columbus, where we just had a much smaller Wild Oats store, though it did serve my needs there. It was nice to have a much larger selection of grains, nuts, seeds, packaged goods, meat and dairy products free of pesticides and hormones, baked goods, vitamins, and more. Whenever I went, careless neighbors clamored for a seat in my car.

I had brought along a laptop computer to keep up with my workplace through e-mail. I ate three meals a day in the apartment, while reading e-mail and news on the Internet. That also allowed me to be in frequent communication with my colleagues, and sometimes do a few things on the computers back home.

It was the plan to be away for four weeks, but it crept up to seven weeks. Despite the slow network connection, I could do enough work from there to keep my customers happy. Combined, I logged in a full workweek while there.

We did have a long weekend where a customer converted to a new computer system that was to be managed by someone else. This hand-over had been delayed many times, which in turn had delayed my trip to Dallas for months. It was considered to fly me back to Columbus for a few days; I was very glad that was not necessary. Airplanes have extremely poor air quality inside, so it would have made me sick for days, even while wearing a mask.

There were many interesting neighbors. Right next door was a nurse from Germany, who shared the apartment with a doctor from New York. There was also an executive from China, a wonderful lady who every morning would stand in the grassy courtyard and do her Chi-Gong exercises.

Then there was a mechanic from Canada, who considered it a good night if he slept two hours. I watched in amazement how he, in just a month, came to sleep a regular eight hours a night and changed from a silent man to a happy man. He called up his doctor back in Canada, who refused to believe that the change was possible.

Another patient was a woman who had arrived with her hands nearly black from scleroderma, facing possible amputation. When I first met her, her hands were still white as a sheet, but when she flew home, they were already pinkish. She had mercury fillings in all her teeth (dentists call them amalgams), which she would have to get removed, or she would soon again see her hands turn black. Dr. Rea knew a holistic dentist in her home state who knew how to remove amalgams safely, so she would not get further poisoned during their removal.

I enjoyed being in a community of people who understood things. One simply has to have this illness to be able to understand how deeply it changes one's life, and how to be "safe" to be around. We shared a bond of understanding, perhaps like people who have gone through military training or came from the same foreign country. It was liberating that I could just walk up to other people and not be concerned about whether they would make me sick.

I was suddenly able to have a social life again. We had several get-togethers in the evenings, sometimes even with guests from the permanent community in Dallas.

People were generally very friendly. I made a remark about that to a Canadian woman I had spent some time with, and she replied that a lot of the women here were friendlier to me than to other women! I had not considered that, but she was right. At least two-thirds of the patients were women, and most in my age group. It seems that our bodies start to break down against the chemical onslaught around age 35 to 45, though I have seen patients from around a year old and well into their eighties.

Why there is such a majority of women with this disease, nobody knows, but there are many other illnesses with gender imbalances, some even more so.

When I looked around room "B" at the clinic, I realized that few people were married. This illness is a real marriage breaker; not many spouses can deal with the level of change we have to go through. The spouses who do hang on are the unsung heroes of this illness, as it is often a thankless job to provide financial and emotional support, as well as most of the chores that the sick person can no longer do. The spouse will have to clean up their lives as thoroughly as the sick person, and cannot check him or herself whether that trip to the store contaminated the clothes enough to be a problem for the sensitive spouse.

I have never been much for the artificial look of the American Woman, as glorified by many magazines which aim to make women feel bad about themselves, so they go and buy these expensive, and often very unhealthy beauty products. At this clinic, very few women wore any kind of make-up; most didn't even color their hair. No fancy clothes either; it was typically plain cotton clothes. People who are familiar with us can often spot an EI. Plainness is our uniform.

There was a woman whom I shall refer to as Tina. The poor woman had bipolar disorder, also called manic-depressiveness, and she had entered a manic phase. It was thought that her behavior changes were caused by environmental exposures, so Dr. Rea suggested to her that she try to stay in the cleaner air outside Dallas. He specifically recommended a place near Seagoville, southeast of Dallas. I had heard about the place and was curious to see it. I volunteered to drive her.

It took about an hour to get there, most of it on the freeway. She talked the whole way as if there was no tomorrow. The last miles were along calm country roads to a wooded parking lot in an area that seemed much further from Dallas than it really was. From the parking lot, we had to walk a hundred yards out on a peninsula surrounded by water. Here was a little village of steel huts and aluminum trailers, around a big lawn. It was very different from any other place that I had ever seen before. I recognized two people living there, whom I had met at the clinic.

When we had been there for about 15 minutes, I noticed that Tina didn't say much. She seemed quite normal, engaging in normal conversation. Amazing. I mentioned it to her, and she had noticed it, too. She said she also felt better there than in Dallas. So did I. The outside air was much better. I had no need to wear a mask, like I did whenever outside in Dallas.

Tina decided to move the next day, and I drove her back to Dallas. We had only been on the freeway for a few minutes, when the traffic fumes must have gotten to her, as she again started talking a blue streak and was fidgeting. She really needed to move out there.

I came to visit the place a few times in the following weeks. Once I drove an old man out there. He wasn't doing well in the apartment he shared with the mechanic from Canada, so he wanted to see if Seagoville was better for him. He was a rather bewildered old man, who had a hard time coming to terms with the reality of his illness. He had flown down with his wife, who was not very supportive of him and quickly got tired of Dallas and flew home, leaving him here.

A week later, I drove out to visit Tina with a carload of fellow patients, who wanted to visit her and see this odd place. It had to be on a Sunday, as that was the only day of the week the clinic was closed, even though on that day our warm fall weather turned out to be dark and cold, with temperatures in the 50s and a cold wind coming down from the north. We braved the sudden chill and sat for a couple of hours in the shared kitchen shack. It was a cold metal shack, with no insulation at all and just two electric space heaters to add a few degrees of warmth to the large room. I was glad to return to my warm cozy apartment, glad I didn't live out there.

The idea that people's behavior can be so strongly influenced by environmental factors was new to me, but it really seemed to be the case with Tina. Sure, I am not very chipper when my head feels like the flu is on, or I can get angry at people who can give me such unpleasant symptoms, just because they like to lather themselves up with fragrances or light up a cigarette, but that is understandable. It is also understandable enough that people who don't know they are chemically sensitive, and live in unhealthy situations, can be labeled as depressive.

Then I saw a video for sale at the clinic store. It was about how the environment can affect school children, made by Dr. Doris Rapp, a pediatrician in Buffalo, New York (now retired). I bought it and saw it on the TV in my apartment. It was amazing. The program showed several of Dr. Rapp's young patients in her office, before and after they receive an injection of something they are strongly allergic to, such as corn or sugar. The patients range from a baby to a 16-year-old girl who becomes suicidal. The video showed small children first sitting quietly with a coloring book or writing on a sheet. Then after the injection, the child becomes uncontrollable. One young boy hits his mom so hard she screamed.

Several samples of handwriting and drawings before and after are shown. The change is obvious. A neat handwriting changes to a bold, sloppy one; a nice coloring book becomes angrily overdrawn.

The little library in the apartment rental office had a copy of Dr. Rapp's book *Is This Your Child?*, which was interesting — and became the last book I was able to read for more than a year. It would be a mighty good idea if school children were checked out for allergy problems before being labeled with ADD or ADHD and subdued with drugs, but the world is apparently not ready for such heresy yet.

I happened to see the front page of *Wired Magazine* at the newsstand in Whole Foods. It talked about a company that had invented a device to connect to a PC, which could generate any sort of smell desired. I bought the magazine, pulled out the article for offgassing, and then read about this new horror. In my mind, I could see this device being used in movie theaters, store displays, and hooked up to TV sets at home. There are people enough with respiratory illnesses; we do not need any more. I was relieved when a few years later, I learned that the company had gone bankrupt before the product hit the market, but this technology will probably rear its ugly head again.

One woman at the clinic was always dressed nicely, using little hats and white gloves. She told me that she was particularly sensitive to the sun's rays, so she had to protect her skin, or it would get red and blister very quickly. She said that it was a part of her electrical sensitivity. Any sort of electromagnetic radiation is a problem for her. I saw and heard many strange things in Dallas, but that things like TVs, refrigerators, and power lines could be harmful was hard to grasp. I had heard before about a controversy regarding radiation from computer screens, which I was occasionally asked about at work, but there was not much information about it. It didn't seem to be supported by medical researchers, at least not in the computer journals that I read.

Some days later, the woman knocked on my door, and we stood and talked for awhile in the middle of my living room. She then told me that something there bothered her electrically. There was nothing to see. Perhaps something under the floor? She told me we could check with something called a gaussmeter. We could probably borrow one from a patient across the courtyard who was also electrosensitive. We borrowed the instrument, and it was clear that something was going on exactly where she had indicated. The meter showed nothing a foot or two away, but clearly showed something where we stood. I could trace it along the floor and eventually to the breaker box, so there was undoubtedly an electrical wire running under the floor. And she could sense that! Intriguing.

There was another building complex near the clinic, called Raintree Apartments, which had housing for people with environmental illness. Twelve apartments had been modified in a building in the rear of the complex. They were tiny apartments with raw concrete floors, no tiling. Most of these were rented out on long-term leases to people who lived permanently in Dallas, though a couple spaces were available at daily and weekly rates.

Some people had actually moved permanently to Dallas, to be near the clinic, and to find housing that was better than what they could find in their home states.

The managers of the complex were painting the outside of all the buildings and would soon come to this one. The EIs living there pleaded for their building to be left alone, but that was refused. Some of us in Dr. Rea's apartments volunteered to take in refugees for a couple of days while the painting took place, but at the last minute, the building managers relented and left the building alone.

That renovations are a very real threat to us really hit home one evening. I came home and the whole place stunk of tar. Even with the windows closed tightly and the air purifier running, I felt terrible all night. I discovered the culprit the next day: the roof of an apartment building a hundred yards away had just been tarred.

I was interested in seeing what a really safe house looked like, one less austere than those places I had seen so far. We organized tours of three homes for myself and others.

The first was an apartment in the northeast corner of Dallas, where a woman lived by herself. Her apartment looked fairly conventional, except the floor was covered with nice tiles. There was no carpeting, but that is not so unusual in this part of the country. The furniture was simple, with removable cushions, no upholstery. All appliances were electric. The place had a neat look, with no knick-knacks that could gather dust.

Then we saw a house, southeast of Dallas. It looked similar, with tiled floors and all-electric appliances. Some of the bedroom walls were covered with an airtight barrier of aluminum foil, as the previous owners had used so much fragrance in those rooms, that it had become embedded in the drywall and impossible to remove.

The last house we saw was in an upscale neighborhood and was a real showpiece. It did not look "EI" at all, though all materials were healthy. They had to replace the roof when they bought the house, and installed a steel roof instead of the usual tar shingles. The heating system was completely redone, using metal ductwork that had been cleaned to remove oily residues from the manufacturing. A sophisticated filtering system mounted on the furnace made the inside air great, despite being in a very polluted part of Dallas.

The floors were covered with beautiful tiles, while the furniture was modern stylish creations of steel, glass and cotton. Glass sculptures and glass-enclosed paintings decorated the rooms very tastefully. The outside pool had a filtering system that required no use of chlorine.

Tiled floors are the safest alternative to carpeting, and pretty much standard for healthy houses for the really sensitive. It does have some draw-backs, however. It is cold to walk on without shoes in the winter and it is a hard surface to drop things on. I dropped my glasses on the floor in my apartment, and one lens broke. I got the number for a Lenscrafters store in the area and called them up. When I was told they were located inside a covered mall, I asked if there was another store somewhere. When he asked why, I explained my problem about going into stores and that an enclosed mall would increase that problem. He immediately volunteered to come to my apartment that evening, though we settled on meeting in the parking lot outside the mall.

I still had to wear a mask, as he showed up wearing a strong cologne. Even outside, it was so strong that my clothes smelled of it afterwards, so I had to change clothes before going to the clinic. When I met him again to pick up the repaired glasses, he had made sure not to put cologne on that day.

There are really some nice folks in Texas, I must say. He told me that the company had recently sent him to a day of disability awareness training. They were shown a video on how to deal with various situations. One of the shown challenges was helping a person with MCS, so he already knew about us.

After seven weeks, it was time to go home to Ohio again. I had stayed as long as I possibly could and didn't see a need to stay any longer. I could not afford it either, as my insurance plan had told me in advance that they considered the sauna treatment "experimental," and the apartment rent was expensive too.

I packed up to leave for home Saturday before Thanksgiving. I was bringing a stack of frozen allergy vials with me. I had filled a small cooler with water and frozen the vials into a solid block of ice, to keep them frozen as long as possible. The whole cooler was kept in the freezer until I was ready to leave, and then I forgot it. I had already thrown the key in through the mail slot to the rental office when I remembered it. The office would be closed until Monday. The clinic had recently hired a new manager for their apartments. She cheerfully drove there to let me in, so I gave her a big hug and headed for Ohio.

In Texarkana, on the Arkansas border, it was the third gas station I went to that accepted credit cards at the pump; otherwise, it went smoothly. Frosty weather had been promised for central Arkansas, but warmer closer to the Mississippi River, so I tried to get close to it for the night. I was not well equipped for winter camping.

There are not many places to camp in that part of Arkansas. I headed for Village Creek State Park, about 30 miles west of Memphis. It was dark and drizzly when I got to the area, and I could not find the park. I gave up and drove up next to a radio tower that stood by itself, surrounded by a lot of bushes that would hide myself and the car from the road. I spent the night there in my tent.

I was up and on the road again before dawn. It was cold and foggy, no reason to linger. I drove all the way back to Ohio that day. Seven hundred miles, the longest I've ever done. I would consider half that a good day, but another cold night did not appeal to me without more winter gear.

I arrived at my apartment in Columbus around 10:00 P.M., very tired from the long drive. In my seven-week absence, King Mold had taken the opportunity to expand his empire in the bathroom. The apartment also smelled of fresh paint, probably from the new strip mall that was now nearly finished next door. I had to spend some time disinfecting the bathroom and air out the apartment. This helped me get through the night, but it was not a long-term solution.

8

Winter in Ohio

I was quickly back in full swing again, keeping my job afloat while working on the health problems facing me. Within a few days, I located a small local company that rents out industrial-strength ozone machines, to get rid of the mold that had taken over the apartment in my absence. Or perhaps I just noticed it more now, as mold is really always present in a carpeted room.

I picked up the machine Thanksgiving morning. The owner worked out of his basement and didn't mind serving me on this day. The machine was bulky and weighed about forty pounds. It was capable of ozoning a whole house, and was mostly rented by contractors cleaning up after a fire, using the ozone to get rid of the smoke smell.

The owner recommended I use a low setting. I knew there was a danger running the machine too much, as it could permanently make a place stink of ozone, making me homeless. I've heard stories of people who had to sell their house after overdoing it.

I decided to try the bedroom first. I could live without that room if I had to. The machine ran for seventeen minutes, then I ran inside and opened all the windows while I held my breath. I had some work to do at off-hours down on campus, and left for about four hours.

When I came back, the ozone smell had left and the treatment seemed to help. The next weekend, I rented the machine again and ran it for three hours on the whole apartment Sunday morning. While it aired out, I returned the machine and spent the rest of the day in the clean air north of the city.

The apartment was uninhabitable when I returned in the evening. It still reeked of the ozone treatment. The bathroom was pretty good, though, as there were no carpeting or other fabrics to absorb the ozone smell. I camped in there for the night, with an air cleaner, the telephone and an electrical heater.

The next morning, the smell was more tolerable, as long as I kept the windows open. It was only 38 degrees outside, so I had to start my workday wearing a winter coat. Later in the day, I could close up the place again, and now I felt better being there than before, so the whole ordeal had been worth it.

Being a computer person, I too was involved in the big Y2K hullabaloo. The concern was that some computers might cease functioning correctly at the stroke of midnight on New Year's Eve, as they might suddenly think we were in the year 1900, instead of 2000. I had slowly worked on the issue over the past two years, checking our in-house computer software (which only had one real problem) and upgrading computers to what the vendors told me they guaranteed would work. One of the computers will "forever" have the date set at December 31, 1999, so an old database on it could be used for a while longer.

The university started taking this issue very seriously that fall, and even hired a "Y2K czar," who created a big bureaucracy that demanded that I redo a lot of what I had done, just to fill out their endless forms.

The university was closed on December 31, but I went in to copy all data to tape on all the central computers I was responsible for. As I was leaving one building, I noticed the lights were on in a large office landscape. I didn't see anybody, so I turned the lights off. I hadn't noticed a woman in the far end of the room, who shouted out. I turned the lights back on. She stood up and looked at me across the big room. I just waved and walked out.

She noticed I wore a mask and got so afraid she called the police. They arrived in two police cars after I left the building, did a thorough search for this mysterious man, and then left. The woman then called the building manager at home, who figured it was me. The woman was a rather new employee, who had not heard about me.

I was comfortably prepared for the big night. None of the systems under my jurisdiction were on the "critically important" list, so I didn't have to report anything to the "czar's" command center, unless something went really bad. Through my inspections, I had located one possible hazard that wasn't really related to computers, but had to be taken seriously. My customer had a warehouse storing various hazardous chemicals. If we had severe freezing weather, and they lost power for more than about 24 hours, some of the liquids could freeze and break their bottles. The chemicals could then run into the drains in the floor and, somewhere down the line, combine into explosive compounds. To be on the safe side, we had a heated truck on retainer at a local trucking company, and the manager spent the night in the building, playing cards with some friends.

The night was uneventful. America did the transition after most of the world, which had few problems of consequence. As soon as midnight passed, I connected to each of my computers, which all happily accepted the new century.

The new strip mall next door was almost completed. Fortunately, all the painting of the outside walls had been done while I was in Dallas. It would otherwise have required me to leave for several days. The little access road down the side of the building, and right outside my windows, was first surfaced in December. I had to leave during the day they did it. Even the closed windows were not enough to keep the tar fumes away, but it was fine by evening. Had it been during the hot summer, it would have been a problem for at least a week.

I continued hiking every Sunday with a friend. Since it got cooler, we could return to our favorite metro park. We had to switch during the summer, as there were too many highly fragranced joggers that would pass and leave a foul scent-trail behind them that would linger for several minutes. I once saw two joggers really load up with spray cans of fragranced deodorants before hitting the trail. It almost seemed like they were spray-painting their whole body with the stuff! To imagine they just might smell themselves sometime!

My hiking friend was using some sort of fragranced shaving cream that bothered me. I suggested he try to switch to a non-toxic brand, but he preferred simply not to shave on the morning we went hiking. He would also wear the same clothes he wore the day before, so they had aired out some.

I was glad for his weekly company, especially since he was sometimes the only human being I saw during the week. He was a member of a nudist club and had invited me to some of their outings during the summer. I thought that was a good idea, as there would be no clothes loaded with detergents or fabric softeners to make me sick. I went two times. The first time went well. I had a fun day playing volleyball, and could almost be like a normal person for a precious few hours, as long as I steered clear of a few people. When I went again the following year, I had become more sensitive and had a big problem being around most people and their sunscreens, so I had to leave again.

When I returned from Dallas, I generally felt better than before I left. I was still super-extra sensitive, but that quieted down to the level it was before within four weeks. Most importantly, the burning sensation in my head was still gone. It had plagued me every day until I left for Dallas and did not return when I came home again.

But after a couple of months, the benefit of the Dallas trip seemed to evaporate again. It was in the middle of the winter, always my worst time of the year. I would get general headaches again, the burning sensation in my forehead would slowly start to show up in the evenings, then gradually earlier in the day. Next morning, it would always be gone. The only days it didn't show up were Sundays, if I stayed out of town all day. It affected my vision; things would not be sharp, almost unreal, even though my glasses were perfectly matched to my eyes. It felt like the flu was coming on, but it never did, and there was never a fever. It was again difficult to concentrate enough to get anything done, to sort of "burn through" the fog, pain, and cobwebs in my brain.

I normally had lots of physical energy, but sometimes I would get really fatigued and had to drag myself around. That could even happen during our Sunday hike, presumably due to mold or some other problem in the forest.

One thing that didn't improve at all from the Dallas trip was my amazing sensitivity to any sort of printed material, so I worked on going completely paperless, except for note paper and incoming bills. The bills would be aired out on the balcony for a whole day, before I would look at them. Other unavoidable materials would be offgassed the same way, though I sometimes had to save them from rains that could reach in under the little roof covering the balcony.

When I needed to write a check, I had to go out on the balcony, hold my breath, write it out, then hang it on the clothesline and go back inside again. I tried to write them in pencil, but a couple were returned for that reason, and I had to air out the printed check anyway.

I used to subscribe to more than a dozen magazines, most of them related to my work, but they all had to be canceled as I could no longer tolerate them. Except one — one magazine was determined to make their magazine as ecological as possible, using ecological inks and chlorine-free paper. That was the only magazine I could continue to read, though I had to do it outside.

The manuals for the various computer systems had been delivered on CDs for some years already, so that was not a problem. There was hardly anything at work that required the use of paper.

Instead of reading regular books and magazines, I would read them on the computer. The major newspapers and magazines were experimenting with electronic versions on the web, which were free. Two companies had started to sell electronic editions of regular books, but their methods were not fully developed at the time. There were plenty of free books available on the web anyway; most of them older works where the copyright had expired.

I had good use of the borrowed laptop computer for reading and doing some work away from my desk, especially while I ate. I looked for a used one on the Internet, one that was fairly old, so it would have been offgassed. Eventually, I bought one that was three years old from a guy in Florida. He assured me that he did not smoke or use any fragrances, but it still stunk of perfume. The guy apologized that he had let his wife use it recently.

I washed the outside of it, and let it air out. After a month, it was usable, though the electrical cord still stunk. Soft plastic absorbs the stuff better than a hard surface. Even years later, that cord still has a fragrance to it. The nice carrying case that came with the laptop was impossible to clean and had to be thrown out.

My own desktop computer was about four years old and in need of an upgrade. Four years is a long time in this business, though my needs were modest as all the heavy work was done on remote computers, not on the one in front of me. I would not be able to handle a newer computer; even mine still had a slight chemical odor to it coming out from the cooling fan. Computers contain many types of toxic chemicals, such as plastics, epoxies and flame-retarding chemicals, which especially offgas when it gets warm. I kept the window next to the computer open whenever it was on.

I ended up simply upgrading the processor to nearly double the speed, and adding an extra hard drive. This machine was not used for games or video or such things that really required a lot of horsepower.

I had brought a number of allergy vials back from Dallas, which I used to give myself desensitization shots every day. There were also some drops to put under my tongue to desensitize me to colognes and fragrances. They contained the offending substances in extremely small concentration, but after a while, they started to bother me and I had to give up using them. I was astounded when I got so sensitive that I could even smell the small drop hanging from the dropper!

At Dr. Rea's suggestion, I ordered a sauna from a company called Heavenly Heat, which is located in Arizona, of all places. I needed to continue sweating out toxins, a treatment that I had started in Dallas.

The sauna was ordered shortly after I returned to Ohio in late November, but it took three months before it arrived. I had ordered a model with glass walls, glass ceiling and a stainless steel floor. Only the frame and the bench were made of wood, and a type of wood with not much turp. The fresh wood still bothered me, so there would have to be a burn-in period.

The 500-pound wooden crate was delivered to a friend's home in February. It took us a few hours to put all the pieces together and wash them in filtered water. The electrical heater came with a timer so it could be set to turn on up to nine hours in advance. It would then burn for an hour and turn itself off. I rewired the timer to keep the heater on for up to nine hours at a time, so it was easy for my friend to run it to offgas the heating elements and the wood turps. The sauna was basically a space heater for the rest of the winter, though my friend also enjoyed sitting in it at least once a week.

While waiting for my sauna to get ready, I shopped around for a used exercise bike to use in the detox program. I found an old ugly one for only $31. It had no smell, but I still had to use it outside on the balcony, as the brake quickly got hot and stinky.

My brother told me that one of his colleagues had a lot of problems with migraine headaches. My brother lent him a copy of the book *An Alternative Approach to Allergies* by Theron Randolph, the initial pioneer of environmental medicine. The man experimented and found out that milk caused his migraines, and now only had one episode per three months. Too bad the guy's doctors didn't think of looking at his diet.

A trip to the dentist went fairly well. I always got the first appointment of the day when I went for a checkup, so I could avoid other patients as much as possible. The staff was very nice not to wear any fragrance that day, and they also reminded the dentist not to lather on his horrible cologne. Of course, his clothes still stunk of cologne. That will never go away, but it was a lot better. He was rather skeptical that it could bother me this much, but he humored me. He also didn't think putting mercury in people's mouths could be harmful, but he was willing to convert a filling or two a year to the more benign, and expensive, gold-platinum alloys. Few dentists are willing to consider the folly of putting a highly toxic metal in people's mouths, but admitting it could probably open them to both legal action as well as a let-down of their egos. The eventual conversion to plastic fillings will happen, but the official reason will surely not be the health benefits.

I decided to try to find a more holistically oriented dentist, if one could be found in Ohio. My present dentist was expanding his practice and moving to a new building. I would not be able to go to him there. Through personal contacts, I got the names of two open-minded dentists. I visited their offices during the winter, but neither place had a good-enough indoor air quality. Both of them had problematic carpeting. It does surprise me that carpeting is even allowed in a health care facility, as they are great breeding grounds for germs.

Every three weeks, I would bake a batch of amaranth "muffins," which were only made from flour, baking soda, olive oil, and the herb Stevia as a sweetener. The grain amaranth is in a different genetic family than the usual grains, so that is a good one to use on a rotation diet.

In her books, Dr. Rogers warns against heating oil to the usual frying temperature as that changes the molecular structure so the oil does not work as well when used in the body's cell membranes. To avoid that, I baked at a low temperature, so it took two full hours in the oven.

I didn't like the smoke coming from the oven, so I would usually go on my weekly shopping run to the Wild Oats store while it baked. One morning when I did that, my beeper went off while I was in the car. I had programmed my main computers to keep an eye on each other and send an e-mail to my beeper if something seemed amiss. That had sometimes allowed me to fix a problem before I would receive a call from the customer. It's always satisfying to inform the customer that the problem has already been taken care of.

This time the beeper message told me that there was a problem with the machine servicing the library system. This computer very seldom had problems, as it was well built with duplicate disk drives and other components.

I continued driving directly to our cavernous main computer room. I was only ten minutes away when the message came in. I located the problem and arranged for repairs that afternoon, which just gave me enough time to hurry home to save the amaranth muffins in the oven. It was hectic to keep up a full-time job and manage this illness.

I would do my weekly shopping trip to Wild Oats on a morning I was not scheduled to work. I went there early to avoid other customers and the cloud of perfumes and fabric softeners that surrounded some, though most of the customers there were health conscious and were fine. It was much worse in other stores, and I rarely went any other place.

Wild Oats had tiled floors and did not use fragrances anywhere, including the restroom. It had only been a fad for a few years to have those automatic fragrance sprays in most restrooms, making them inaccessible to people with MCS.

If I had to go to such a restroom, or most other stores, I had to wear my respirator with charcoal filters and sometimes even had to change my clothes after leaving the store as the stench hung in cotton clothing, making me sick once I took the mask off.

There were times when I even had to wear the mask inside Wild Oats. Occasionally, I would notice a little kid asking mommy about me. Typically the parent would either hush up the child, or just explain that the man over there had allergies. Sometimes, I would take off my mask, smile and explain it briefly to the child. Might as well let the next generation know what they will have to deal with.

I could often guess who was "loaded" with chemicals, just by looking at them, and steer clear of them. It was sort of an MCS profiling system, making sure the women with big hairdos were given a wide berth, along with highly obese women, young women with their boyfriends, older ladies with blue hair, and guys who looked like salesmen.

Within the last year, I started to be able to buy many things over the internet. I used it to buy a lot of small things, like postage stamps and office supplies. I also bought upgrades to my PC there. I rarely needed to go anywhere else than Wild Oats.

The largest newspaper in Arizona, the *Arizona Republic*, printed on March 19, 2000, a nice article about an airline stewardess who had become chemically sensitive and who had to live in a tent in the desert outside Tucson. A month or two later, one of the big network TV stations aired a five-minute interview with her and her doctor. It was nicely done, without the sensationalism so common in the media. I was hopeful that the media would maybe help us gain some much-needed acceptance.

I had heard about a company that made ventilated boxes to put around a computer to vent the fumes to the outside. It didn't seem worth it to buy one of these very expensive boxes for my computer. However, I bought one that was designed for reading materials, called a reading box. It cost about $400 and was very nicely done. They hand-make them in a little shop that employs people with MCS. The box was made of aluminum, with a glass top. It had a hose attached to one side, which went to a powerful fan mounted in the window. The other end of the box is open, but the fan creates a strong wind inside that prevents the fumes from escaping. It was a virtual storm that was so strong it sometimes would turn the pages of a magazine.

To flip the pages, I would stick my hand inside the box through the open side. I quickly learned that when I pulled my hand back out again, it was enough to bring out a tiny amount of air from the box, despite the roaring fan, and enough to irritate my sinuses. The solution was to either keep the hand inside the box while I read, or use a pencil to flip the pages with.

It was nice to be able to read a magazine again, though it was cumbersome and took up the whole table. I could not eat and read at the same time, so I ended up not using the box much, as I had very little time available. I was struggling to keep my job afloat and had to spend extra hours working to make up for the time I lost simply being spaced out. My household chores took up the rest, particularly creating three meals a day from scratch, as well as my all-important walks to get fresh air. I would go for a walk every morning, and sometimes also during lunch and after hours. It helped clear the "cobwebs" that accumulated in my head whenever I was inside. The university had a farm a few hundred yards away, which was an excellent place to go without any nearby traffic or people.

The water quality in Columbus was a problem. The chlorination bothered me, so I had a filter both on the kitchen sink and the shower head. Before I put the filter on the shower head, the air filter in the bathroom would cake up with a white powder. Now it was just regular dust. Glad I didn't have to breathe in all that, even if the powder was probably just calcium.

I realized that my apartment wasn't healthy enough for me, despite getting rid of a lot of problems. The inside was pretty good, but the activities of my neighbors were a daily problem. In the winter, many would run their fireplaces on the weekends, and the smoke was impossible to keep out, even with closed windows.

I had to air out the apartment at least once a day. It would be better to keep the windows open all the time, but I would often get in trouble with fumes rolling in from diesel trucks delivering goods, or the occasional barbecue. The worst problem was the fumes from the neighbors' clothes dryers, especially two women next door who washed their work clothes every day using really toxic stuff. I constantly had to be ready to seal up the place.

I had moved to this apartment three years earlier, because the downstairs neighbor at the other place used her barbecue at least three times a week. There was also a mold problem in the apartment and a wetland right outside.

Cold drafts were also a problem, as they make my head hurt for some reason. That had always been a problem, especially when for a time I shared an office with a colleague who loved to wear sweaters in the summer, so she kept the place really cold with a cold draft coming out the register above my head.

It's a job making a home healthier. My apartment was twelve years old, which is about the minimum amount of time for outgassing the formaldehyde in the walls, floors, and cabinetry. I had taken the kitchen cabinets apart and sealed all the surfaces to contain the remaining turps and formaldehyde. The fireplace was sealed off, too, to prevent soot from coming down the chimney.

The carpet was the original. Not pretty, but old. But old carpets store a lot of dirt and usually contain mold, so I was advised to get rid of it. It is simply not possible to clean a carpet, no matter what. Years later, I had a discussion about that with a professional carpet cleaner who got MCS. He was absolutely convinced he could make his own carpet completely clean, using some super-effective machinery. Well, eventually I talked him into pulling up one corner of his now extremely well cleaned carpet — he was astounded to discover how much dirt was still there.

I talked with my landlord about removing the carpet in my apartment. He was very supportive and even offered $500 towards the cost of tiling the place, but I could not use ceramic tiles. He didn't think the floor could hold the weight, and it would not be possible to install a new carpet over the tiles. In Ohio, it would be impossible to rent out the place again if there was no carpet.

After much searching, I did find some thin lightweight tiles made of a natural material, resembling linoleum. They were produced by a company in Quebec, Canada, from their factory in France. They had to be special ordered and shipped by boat, so it would take months for them to arrive.

A colleague from work offered to install the tiles, with me as his assistant. He gave me samples of the material he uses to glue the tiles with, and it seemed fine once it had cured.

While I waited, I ordered a roll of K-Shield (similar to Denny foil), which is strong paper with aluminum foil on both sides. This was used to cover the floor in the bedroom, the most important room in the house. If the body is not given proper rest from irritants during the night, there is little hope of a recovery.

I also used some of the foil to cover the insides of the furnace, which had a lot of mineral wool insulation exposed to the airflow.

Two big air cleaners arrived by mail from Dallas. They were expensive at $360 each, but state of the art, with 15 pounds of charcoal and zeolite filter material in each. I gave my older filter to a friend, whose wife had asthma.

I also bought a big dehumidifier, to keep down the humidity during the muggy Ohio summer, which should also help on the mold problem. It stunk terribly when it ran, as there was some disgusting insulation material around some of the piping in it. I ran it outside for several days, hoping it would offgas, but eventually I had to return it.

I thought about moving, but it is difficult to find something better. Any apartment would likely have had the carpet cleaned and the walls painted, so it would be uninhabitable for many months. A house of my own would be better, but I was very reluctant for such a potentially expensive adventure. I talked with a fellow patient who lived a hundred miles west of Columbus. Her two daughters were attending the university and had rented an older house near the campus. The older daughter was also sensitive but did well in their rented house. She was graduating and moving out, while the younger daughter would move to some student housing. They were very nice to let me visit and see how I did in the house. I seemed fine on that warm day in the early spring, and I was very close to signing a lease, when Dr. Rea talked me out of it. He basically told me that none of his patients had ever recovered while living in a house heated with gas, like this one was. Even an old leaky house.

I didn't have my own washing machine, but used a laundromat across the street on Sawmill Road. It was a small place, run by a Korean family. I had enough clothing that I only needed to go over there once every three weeks. I would be there when they opened up in the morning, so I pretty much could be done before there were other customers stinking up the place. In the summer I would only wash the clothes, then hang them up to dry at home. In the winter, I also had to use their clothes dryers.

In mid–March, I did such a laundry run, which turned into a disaster. I think the previous user of the clothes dryer must have used dryer sheets, which had coated the inside of the drum with their chemicals, and then transferred the chemicals to my clothes when I used it. All my clothes got contaminated by fabric softener, which is one of the things I was the most sensitive to. When I came home with this enormous pile of clothes and hung them up, I got really sick from it. I sought to control the contamination by sealing all the clothes up in plastic trash bags, and from then on only using three sets of clothes that I would wash in the bath tub. I assumed I would recover after a few days, but not this time.

Once every few years, someone tries a new alternative treatment and gets healed. The story quickly travels around and many patients jump on the bandwagon, hoping this is finally the cure. Over a year or two, it seems that every other patient is trying the new treatment of the day. Some report improvements, further fueling the interest, but eventually the excitement fades. The treatment then enters the long list of "occasionally works" treatments.

While I was in Dallas, I heard stories about a new treatment system I will refer to as the Next Great Thing. After I returned to Ohio, I kept in contact with one person who was being treated with the Next Great Thing. She felt it was helpful and when she reported that she could now read books again, I decided to try it too.

I looked around for alternative health practitioners in central Ohio and found a Next Great Thing practitioner, whom I shall refer to as Dr. Q.

Dr. Q was a very likeable man, and he was familiar with MCS. He had one other patient with MCS, whom I talked to a few times over the phone. She was living in her bathroom, as that was the only part of the house she could be in. The rest of her house was too toxic after they had new carpeting and new furniture installed, which her husband refused to take out again.

Dr. Q started by testing me for what I was allergic to.

The testing method is called kinesiology, or "muscle testing." He gave me a sample of some substance, that I should hold in my left hand. Then I held my right arm straight out from my body. He then pressed down on my arm, to see how strong it is. If I am allergic to what is in the sample, it weakens my muscles, and he can easily press my arm down. It is a method to bypass the conscious mind, to ask questions directly, and though it did seem rather strange, it did seem to work as he tested me with various compounds and got the responses that were expected. I decided to keep an open mind.

Dr. Q then used the treatment samples. After each treatment I had to avoid the substance completely for a while. For example, when I was treated for chicken, I could not eat chicken or eggs, nor could I sleep with my down comforter. There are several alternative treatments that use this general method.

Like most alternative treatments, the Next Great Thing takes a lot of sessions to have an effect. It works more gently, by nudging the body to accept a substance as harmless again. We did two sessions a week for months.

The treatments seemed to work, as I started to eat chicken, eggs, rice, wheat, and oats again. I cautiously started eating them to see if they caused any problems, then gradually worked them into my four-day rotation diet. It was now 16 months since Dr. Rogers took them off my diet. Whether the treatments did it, or it simply was time to start using them again anyway, I don't know. In any case, they were a much welcome addition.

Later I noticed that I was a little less sensitive to fragrances and dryer exhaust from the neighbors. I used to be so sensitive that a single breath from the scent-trail left by a passing fragrance user was a problem. That little was enough to get my sinuses to burn for hours and make my mind unclear, as if it only ran at half speed. Sometimes I would take a "hit" from people I couldn't even see, like when the breeze was just right and the fragrances were carried for a hundred yards or more.

Now I was suddenly able to tolerate three or four breaths of this toxic drift, before my sinuses would flare up. That was a tremendous improvement, as one breath of the stuff would be enough to alert me to hold my breath and move away. It was already an automatic response for me to hold my breath as soon as I detected any chemical odor. I didn't have to think about it.

I assumed the reason I could not tolerate more than a few breaths was that the stuff is still quite toxic, and the Next Great Thing only works on the allergic-type responses. This is only my own guess, though.

The treatment also helped with the dryer exhausts that on many calm evenings enveloped the apartment building in a toxic cloud. I was now able to tolerate more of that as well, so I could safely go in and out of the building by just holding my breath.

We were clearly onto something here. I was very optimistic. There was now a light in the dark tunnel, and it didn't look like an oncoming train. I was wrong.

9

The Day the World Changed

Monday April 17, 2000, was a long day. My job duties allowed me to move my work time around quite a bit, and my work hours regularly included evenings. I could do almost everything from home, but one or two nights a week I would drive to the campus, put on my respirator and take care of various things with the computers, pick up mail, make photocopies, etc. I did this in the evening to be undisturbed. Some of the work also required that nobody was using the central computer or network.

I had been in the building for a few hours and was doing the last item on my to-do list, a minor adjustment to the assistant director's desktop PC. I noticed that his large CRT screen was a little fuzzy, which could be caused by a magnetization of the perforated metal plate that sits inside the monitor, right behind the glass plate. It can slowly build up over time, and mostly happens with large CRT computer monitors. It's easy to fix by engaging the "degaussing button," which for a few seconds applies a very strong magnetic field to the screen. As soon as I pressed the button, it felt like I was hit on my forehead. I could feel a burning sensation there, the same burning sensation that had plagued me for over a year. It had been really bad the previous summer and was a big reason I had to give up my office in this building. Though I didn't know the cause of it, this burning headache would start within minutes of entering the office, while at home it tended to first start during the day. Until recently, it would first happen in the evenings at home, then gradually earlier in the day. And not at all if I went for a walk in the park on Sunday. It now made sense. Whenever I was home, the computer would be on from when I woke up until I went to bed. I used it for everything now, as I could not handle printed materials because of my extreme ink sensitivity. My campus office had two PCs and a network server. There was also an electrical transformer mounted on the other side of the wall, about five or six feet from my chair. This transformer steps down a high voltage to ordinary 110 volt.

I had borrowed a laptop computer from a colleague to bring on the trip to Dallas. Shortly before the trip, I tried to use it in my car, with it sitting on my lap. That quickly became uncomfortable, both from the heat but also from a strange sensation in my legs that I now recognize, but then didn't consider further. When I used the laptop in Dallas, I had no problems simply because I only used it for an hour or two each day, and a laptop's flat screen emits less radiation than a CRT computer monitor.

Well, I've been able to work my way around all the other problems that environmental illness had thrown at me, so I will conquer this one as well. At least now I knew what caused these burning head pains. It was the electromagnetic radiation! The next morning, I didn't turn on any computer, as I wanted to give myself a break from it.

I drove to my appointment with a medical lab in a western suburb of Columbus. Dr. Rea had ordered two new blood tests and a test of my immune system, to see if there was any improvement.

Drawing on my personal contacts, I was able to locate a small private lab that would do it. The two lab technicians were very nice and had been briefed by my friend that my needs were a bit unusual. Their skilled hands quickly got the vials filled. The immune test was more complicated, as they had never seen it before, but the instructions were clear, and I had seen it done before in Dallas.

I drove directly to the campus from the lab. I parked my car in a remote corner of the agricultural section and ate my lunch, before continuing to a monthly meeting with a customer. We normally hold these meetings at the customer's office, but I was unable to be there, so everybody was nice to do it in the large meeting room in my manager's office building. The air quality in that building was not good. I had not been able to work there for several years, but the largest meeting room had a separate ventilation system that is designed for perhaps 30 or 40 people, and there is no carpeting. I can sit well away from our customers, who are usually mildly fragranced, while my manager sits next to me, as she is quite safe.

This time we had to hold the meeting in a smaller meeting room, as the larger one was needed for something else. There was also an extra guest, who was rather fragrant, so I had to put on my mask. Rather that than not being fully coherent, and nobody seemed to take notice. Of course I waited too long to do it, so the rest of the afternoon I was not worth much. At least I could then continue to stay away from computers for the rest of the day, giving my new-found sensitivity a rest. It seemed to work; the burning sensation had not started.

Eating dinner at home made me feel better, as food gives my body more energy. Again, no computer and thus nothing to read during the meal.

I had completely avoided using a computer all day, and at no time had I felt the burning sensation in my head. It had been my daily companion for many months, to the point where I could hardly stand it any longer.

The next morning, I turned on my computer and started reading my e-mails. I was soon rewarded with the familiar burning sensation and realized I was in deep trouble now. It was worse than ever. Perhaps the strong exposure to that degaussing monitor in the office had made it worse. I was now sure I had the dreaded electromagnetic hypersensitivity, EHS, that I had heard about in Dallas.

Discouraged, I went back to bed and laid for hours thinking about my career that was really taking off, and now seemed to have run into an unmovable roadblock. What on earth was I going to do now?

In the afternoon, my fighting spirit came back. I would fight this new problem with all I had, no surrender until forced to do so. I had gotten through a tough engineering school and numerous crises at work by thinking my way out of them, or forcing my way through them, working around them, bridging them, or tunneling under them. I did not give up on things and had always gotten to the other side of an important problem. I made a living solving problems; I should be able to solve this one.

That was probably the worst decision of my life.

First step was to call a colleague, who had lent me his laptop computer, asking for an Ethernet network card for it, so I could connect it to my network service at home instead of using my regular CRT computer. I knew the flat screen of a laptop emits a lot less radiation than a traditional CRT screen.

Meanwhile, I moved my screen five feet away from me, and used the disability settings in Windows 98 to enlarge the part of the screen I was currently working on. The feature is made for people with very poor eyesight and is cumbersome to use, but it was workable. My eyes were burning from the strain, but I was in business again. The radiation-induced burning in my head would first come after using the computer for a couple of hours now.

The network card arrived two days later, and I could switch over to use the laptop instead of my PC. That worked as well as sitting five feet from the other monitor, but it still gave me symptoms after awhile.

A colleague had meanwhile used a cheap gaussmeter to measure how much degaussing that monitor radiated. The scale only went to 30 milli-Gauss, and it topped that, so it was pretty powerful.

To further lower my exposures to electromagnetic fields, I removed all electrical devices around me. There were a lot down by my feet. A power strip had a surge protector in it, which generated some radiation. So did the little plug-in transformer cubes that powered my network connection, answering machine, etc. There was also a battery backup system, so my computer would keep running if there were glitches or outages in the electrical grid. It radiated a lot, so did a couple other things sitting down there. All this stuff was moved to the "electrical ghetto" in the corner of the room, about six feet away from me. I figured that ought to be plenty of distance. Little did I know.

Finally, I put an external keyboard and mouse on the laptop, so I could move it back a little. I had been using a touch pad instead of a mouse for several years, as it was better for my wrist, but now it felt like little electrical shocks to touch the surface.

All this helped, but it was still not enough. The burning in my head still showed up; it was just later in the day. And day by day, it started happening earlier and earlier again. I was in a race that I was still not winning.

Then I could no longer use the telephone. My ear had felt warm while I used it for several weeks, but now it felt like little needles were poked into the ear canal shortly after I put the phone to my ear. I was able to get hold of a really good speakerphone through a friend at the university, and that solved the problem. I could only feel it if I sat a couple of feet from it and had a long conversation. Presumably, it was the electromagnet in the speaker that caused the problem.

The phone was so good that I could stand way back from it and still be heard clearly. It became my lifeline, as my health continued to deteriorate. I got excellent help and encouragement from two fellow patients who had electrosensitivity themselves. On their suggestion, I hooked up my refrigerator to a power strip, so I could turn it off before walking up to it. I used the same setup to cook on an electrical hotplate, turning it off before tending the pot.

My electrical shaver turned out to emit a very strong electromagnetic field — not surprising since a strong magnet makes the blade move back and forth. I started letting my beard grow on days I didn't need to go anywhere, while looking for a better model on the Internet. I found one with a small motor instead, but when it arrived, it was just as bad. I had pretty much settled on growing a beard anyway, as using a blade had other problems, and I had problems enough.

My electrosensitive friend in Canada sent me a much better gaussmeter, which was more sensitive and accurate than my cheap model. It's amazing how much radiation comes out of ordinary electrical gadgets.

Both fellow EHS sufferers encouraged me to try grounding myself.

During my trip to Dallas I saw people stand in the courtyard without shoes on, sometimes even holding on to the branch of a bush or the trunk of a tree. Now it was my turn. I felt rather silly standing on the grass, just wearing my socks, but whatever it takes. I didn't feel anything from it, but kept doing it every day.

A friend owned a farm in Amish country north of Columbus. I often drove up there to visit and spend the day in the fresh air. One Sunday I brought along the laptop I had bought on eBay to replace the borrowed one. It came without any software on it, so I hooked the computer up to the car's cigarette lighter and began installing Windows 98SE, the most current version at the time. The computer was lying on the ground; I only stepped close when I needed to do anything.

During the lengthy periods when the computer was working, I walked around the woods. As I stood in one place and held on to a branch of a tree, I suddenly felt a tingling in my arm, followed by an amazing sensation. It was almost like my arm was hollow and stuff attached to the inside was being pulled down through my arm and out the hand. My body had now learned to ground itself to the tree, through my arm.

I continued to ground myself daily. Most of the time, I would now feel a pleasant tingling sensation, which would stop after some minutes. That presumably meant I was done. The amazing sensation on this day in early May was never repeated though.

My new sauna had now been running at my friend's house for three months, and a lot of the wood turps had been offgassed. He also wouldn't keep on running it in the summer, as it heated up the house. And I was anxious to continue my sauna therapy, hoping it might help with my electrical problems.

We took it apart and moved it to my bedroom. I used an electrical drill to do the screws, but had to let him do the rest as my hand got burning hot from the strong field of the electrical motor.

Now I finally had my sauna, and could continue the treatment to remove the solvents and other chemicals stored in my body's fatty tissues. I dearly hoped it might help on the electrical sensitivity, too.

The walls and ceiling in the sauna are glass, while the floor is stainless steel. Only the bench and the frame are wood. It is heated by a 2100 watt electrical heater, which obviously could not be on while I was inside.

We wrapped the whole sauna in Reflectix insulation material, which is basically "bubble wrap" with aluminum foil on both sides—nice material to work with, and pretty inert. Then the sauna would stay hot while I was in it, after turning the heater off.

I used the sauna a least once daily for the next two months, but it did not improve my sensitivities.

I went for walks once or twice a day across the nearby fields. Here the air is cleaner, except for the occasional business jet taking off from the small airfield there. There are no people exuding fragrances or detergent residues, and the cows were certainly no problem.

Sometimes I would lie on the lawn in front of my apartment for grounding, but that was not enough. I ordered a copper bracelet, which I connected with the kitchen faucet through an electrical wire. That didn't do much either, but I could sense a slight tingling when I hooked it up. I also experimented with placing an aluminum plate under my chair, connecting it to the grounding wire, and then placing my bare feet on it while working on the computer. Later I enhanced the grounding by pulling a wire out the window, down a pole and connecting it to a grounding rod.

I took the cabinet of my now-unused PC apart and used the steel plates as shielding material around my laptop, so only the screen was uncovered.

The pain continued. It was like a really bad sinus infection. It wasn't just the burning pain, but it also affected my ability to think clearly. It took a great effort to "burn through the fog," and I often found myself just staring at the screen in a daze. My work suffered tremendously.

It seemed that each new way I thought of to lower my EMF exposure was soon countered by increased sensitivity. It was a tug-of-war, and I was losing ground fast, but I held out, hoping I would finally win with a big techno-fix: a new low-radiation flat LCD computer screen. When I bought the existing monitor two years before, I had looked at the first flat screens that came out but decided not to buy one, as the quality of the picture was not good enough, and they cost about $1,600. The second generation of these screens was coming out now, but they were not yet available in the stores. I did not have time to wait for that, so I decided to buy one unseen. It had gotten good reviews in the computer magazines, and I had used and recommended their products for years. The price was a steep $1,000, but I was able to get one on the eBay on-line auction for $790. It just took awhile to get it delivered. When it finally came, I put it outside on the balcony for a few days so a little of the smell of plastic, flame retardants, and such could gas off. Normally, I would have left it there for weeks, but I did not have time for that luxury. I hoped open windows would be enough; otherwise, I would have to work wearing a respirator.

I decided to try it out after my weekly shopping trip on Thursday, May 18. I drove in to the local Wild Oats supermarket in the morning. The trip went well, except when I passed the row of freezers. They induced a strange tightness in my whole body. That had not happened before, another sign that I was getting worse.

When I came back home, I still had some time before my regular workday started at noon and spent it setting up the safest computer configuration I could. Then I would later set up my workspace from what I learned.

I put all the components on the living room floor, spaced out as far as the extra-long cables would allow. First came the keyboard and mouse; then a couple feet behind them was the new screen. The cables stretched further back to where the computer itself and various extras were placed, in the other end of the living room. I covered the cables with steel plates to deflect radiation away from me.

With all these preparations, I confidently turned it all on — and was thoroughly disappointed. This setup was worse than what I was doing with the laptop!

After convincing myself that this was not workable, I moved all the equipment into a corner, and turned on my laptop to get going with my work. I always started the workday by checking my e-mails, but after just five to ten minutes, I suddenly felt a pain in my chest and then that my esophagus was closing on me.

Scared by this sudden and strong response, I ran out of the room. After calming down for a minute, I ran back in and killed the laptop. No graceful shutdown. Still rather upset, I walked across the parking lot and was lucky to find my friend John at home. He also worked from home parts of the week. I really needed to talk to someone. For the first time in my career, I stared at serious defeat where it mattered. There was no more rope left. I knew I had lost.

I left a phone message to my manager, that things were not going well, and I would not be able to work for awhile. She knew well about my chemical problems, but I had not told many about my new electrical problems. Only a month had passed since I discovered that I was electrosensitive.

The next day I had an appointment with Dr. Q. I had stopped the treatments once I discovered this new problem. One thing at a time. He suggested that we try his Next Great Thing treatment for electrosensitivity. I was treated in his office, and then drove home again. As I had to avoid EMF radiation for the next 25 hours, I had decided to confine myself to a corner of the living room that had the lowest radiation level, according to my gaussmeter. Only the balcony on the other side of the sliding glass door was better, but the weather didn't cooperate.

It was a very boring 25 hours, as I could not read anything, nor go for a walk or talk on the phone. When the time was up, I eagerly tested myself to see how much it had helped. Nothing. No improvement at all.

It was now Saturday, and I had to wait until Monday morning. I first had a phone appointment with Dr. Rea in Dallas. Then I called Dr. Q. He could see me again the next day.

When it was time for my appointment, I went out to my car and started the engine. I could immediately sense a warmth in my left foot, but ignored it and drove off. It kept getting hotter. It was not far to Dr. Q's office; I figured I could do that. But after a couple of miles, the foot felt like it was aflame, and it became unbearable, so I drove off the road and turned off the engine. The burning diminished but did not go away. After a few minutes, I hurried back home. I called Dr. Q, and he promised to come over in a few hours. He did, and treated me again.

I turned off all breakers for the apartment, including the refrigerator. I had prepared myself with foods that did not need to be cooked. I did not have much hope, but it should be tried. There was nothing to lose. It didn't help.

I had asked my friend John to come over shortly after the 25-hour treatment period was over. I asked him to copy some files from my computers to a diskette and then print them out for me. He also connected to the larger computers at work that I managed, and stopped various automatic programs I had set up to keep me informed about their status and send me e-mails, which I could no longer read.

Finally, he typed in and transmitted a message to everybody I used to communicate with by e-mail, briefly describing the situation and that I could no longer be reached by e-mail.

He started doing this on my PC with the flat screen, but that bothered me too much — even when standing 10–12 feet away. Though he does the same kind of work as myself, I still had to be there to guide him through some parts, give him the appropriate passwords, etc. He switched to use the laptop computer, and finished the tasks there, though eventually I still got the now-familiar symptoms in my chest and had to retreat out onto the balcony, sixteen feet from the laptop. We then sat and talked on the balcony for a couple of hours. It was good to discuss this with a friendly, thoughtful person.

About an hour after he left, the situation got out of hand. My neighbors started to come home and turn on their TV's, microwaves, and who knows what. Walls and floors do not stop EMF radiation at all, just like they do not stop radio waves from reaching a TV, radio, or cell phone.

My body picked up all these emissions and I started to have all these terrible symptoms again, including the chest pains, and burning sensations — my whole body was burning now, very painful. I was stunned, didn't know what to do. I was on the threshold of panic when the phone rang. I did not intend to pick it up — a social conversation was not welcome now — but somehow I felt very strongly compelled to answer it, and I did.

It was a healer from Dallas. I had heard about her from some of the electrosensitive people I had talked with. One of them had been greatly helped by her and encouraged me to contact her. I was very skeptical about what a "healer" could do for me, especially from a thousand miles away, but as I continued to get worse, I was willing to try anything. I had called and left her a message some days ago, and again that morning.

I later learned that she couldn't get my number from the first message. The guy who had encouraged me to contact her was on the list of the distress e-mail that John sent out for me that afternoon. When he received it, he contacted her, urging her to call me. So here she was.

I was rather frantic when she called, but her warm voice calmed me, while we talked about what was going on. She then told me she was transmitting to me and asked if I could feel anything unusual.

I focused on myself and was surprised that my symptoms were greatly diminished, my body didn't feel on fire any more. Instead, there was a strange tingling in my feet. Since my ill-fated attempt to drive to Dr. Q's office, I had now and then noticed a tingling in my left foot, the same foot that was burning in the car, but this was different. Pleasant.

The tingling slowly expanded, moving up both my legs, soon encompassing my entire body. It was like standing in a wave of sorts. A stream that seemed to come up from the floor and disappear through the ceiling above my head. It felt very pleasant and peaceful, not at all disturbing. Fascinating. I had never experienced anything remotely like this before.

She told me that somehow, she could "see" me. That I was "all over the place." We talked for about twenty minutes, then she told me she would continue to work on me now, and in the following days she and some apprentices would do some more. I should just take some time now and then and not do anything, especially not read anything, and just let this happen.

She told me her name was Debby and that I should call her again in a few days. She hung up and left me standing in this mysterious wave of energy, in the middle of my living room.

I just kept standing there, letting myself be bathed in this wondrous phenomenon that mocks my years in engineering school. I now knew there was a lot more to human life than what is within the current scientific world view. My world view had suddenly expanded; I knew the frontiers of life were much further away than I had thought.

After a while, I wanted to sit down. But, would I lose this "connection" if I moved across the room? Would this phenomena follow me, or was it fixed in space? If I stepped out of the "beam," could I get back in again? To be safe, I sat down on the floor where I was standing. Eventually I laid down there. The waves continued to roll over me, from the feet up through my body, and I continued to feel a great sense of relief. There was hope now. I was not going to die.

The waves sometimes seemed to sputter and then would pick up again. Meanwhile I just relaxed and let it happen. I once got the thought that maybe it works both ways, and concentrated on the phrase "thank you." Suddenly "you're welcome" appeared in my mind. Was that my own imagination?

After about three hours, it died down and then completely stopped. I sat up and wondered if it was all real. Then I discarded my ruined dinner, I had no interest in food now, and called my friend in Canada who had been helpful with suggestions in the past month. Then I went to bed.

The next morning, things were like the previous morning. I kept wondering whether this was some dream, but each time I concluded it was real enough. I thought of what had happened and likened it to an old cowboy movie with the arrival of the Texas cavalry just in the nick of time to save the pioneers in their Conestoga wagons that were set on fire.

After lunch, I went for a long walk. As I came back and walked into the parking lot of the apartment complex, I could feel the electrical radiation from the motors in all the air conditioners that were now straining against the afternoon heat. Not good.

I realized that I had only been given a short respite, not a miracle. I could no longer stay in my apartment. I quickly went in and packed my tent and a few other things in my backpack and headed into the woods next door. The woods are about fifty acres of dense road-less forest. It is closed to the public, but they would probably forgive me for trespassing, if they ever found out.

It was around 4:00 P.M., so I had to hurry jumping the fence so none of my neighbors returning from work would see me. I found a nice secluded spot and put up the tent. Perfect weather for camping too. The wind did carry some air pollution from the apartments—smoke from grills and exhaust from clothes dryers—but manageable, and it soon died down.

With the tent set up, I laid myself on the ground and immediately felt a lighter version of that "wave" sensation from the night before. I stayed on the ground all evening, and when it was time for bed, I omitted my usual foam pad to sleep closer to the ground. The pleasant tingling "wave" lulled me to sleep.

The sensation was still there the next morning, though barely perceptible. I felt better and had hopes that this would just be another crisis that I would get through and be back to work again in a few days.

It took two years before I had enough understanding to ask more specific questions about what happened that night when "the cavalry" arrived from Texas and pulled me out of the situation. What I then learned was that had Debby not intervened, it was likely that I would have died. If not that evening, then soon after. Without help, the electrical system that governs my body — any body — would have become so overloaded that it would have shut down. The life force would simply have run out of me. In all likelihood, my heart would have stopped. This is the opinion of three people who look at these things from various perspectives and are highly qualified, so I had to accept that. It was typical of Debby not to tell me, but she confirmed it when I asked.

I do know one fellow electrosensitive who did die, but was revived. He had a near-death experience, very similar to those described in the classic book *Life After Life* by Raymond Moody, M.D.

Even though my decision to tough it out to the end did not kill me, it did make me even more sensitive to electrical emissions than I would have been if I had been more sensible and stopped at an earlier point. That month of battling against my own body cost me dearly.

In the previous couple of years before these events, before the burning sensations became such a problem, I noticed another thing that makes me think I was electrically sensitive much earlier. I often had trouble getting going in the morning, feeling tired and unfocused, but once I got going on the computer, I seemed to do better. I learned to depend on this effect, like a coffee drinker on the morning jolt. I thought it was some sort of psychological mechanism that took my attention away from my symptoms, and there was probably some of that as well. But much later did I discover that exposure to EMF can also have a stimulatory effect, which can be very strong. I have since watched myself and others become restless and agitated from electrical exposures, like teenagers on a sugar high.

10

Camp Secret

Spending a night on the ground in the woods seemed to throttle down my hypersensitivity to EMF a bit. It felt calm inside the apartment when I went there to eat my breakfast.

I was concerned about being discovered, so I took great care nobody saw me jump the fence from the woods. Who knows how long I might need to camp in there. It was now the day before the Memorial Day weekend, so people might be home with their TVs and computers turned on, unless I was lucky and they would go someplace else for the long weekend.

I had tried several times the previous day to call the friend who had a farm in Amish country in northern Ohio, but he was hard to get hold of. The next morning he called and told me that the field nearby had just been sprayed with pesticides and that his son was going to have a big bonfire party where I would be camping. The weather forecast was also promising thunderstorms all weekend long. So no trip to the country for now.

My boss had volunteered to drive me up there, and even Dr. Q. would come up to try to treat me one more time in an area where there was absolutely no EMF, so I could stay completely free of it for the requisite 25-hour waiting period. I was disappointed, but maybe it would be possible later.

My immediate needs were taken care of. My boss had arranged a shopping circle, so coworkers would take turns bringing me groceries from the Wild Oats store once a week. That was a great relief. It was interesting to see who stepped forward to help and who didn't. I was surprised several times.

I spent Friday night camping on my balcony, which seemed the safest place that night. The weather wasn't nice, so the air conditioners didn't run and nobody was grilling any food. It only rained a little that night, but Saturday night and all through Sunday it poured down. The soil in the woods was flat and poorly drained, so it turned into a swampland. I did fine in my tent on the covered balcony and was mighty glad I didn't get caught in the morass in the forest.

My friend John came over with a set of e-mail responses to the distress message he sent out to a lot of people for me a few days before. The replies were mostly from other people with environmental illness and carried words of understanding and encouragement. Only one responded back that I must have gone off the deep end. It was from a healthy person. Another healthy person said it must be like being buried alive.

John bought my two-year-old 17-inch computer screen off me, and I gave him an older 15-inch screen. I would only use my new low-radiation flat panel screen once I was able to work again, and I could use the money.

It's good to have such friends next door, but John was moving to a new house a few days later.

Another friend came Tuesday morning and drove me to a K-Mart store about five miles away. It was my first time in a car since I could no longer drive myself. I sat in the back seat, away from the electronics up front. I could still feel my left foot getting warm, but it did not burn. The return trip went even better. That was encouraging. I was concerned I wouldn't be able to tolerate any sort of transportation.

I had a long conversation with Debby in the afternoon. We would talk once a week, while she and two of her apprentices would continue to do their amazing healing work on me.

She told me more about herself. It was interesting to hear that she had to be careful around computers and other sensitive electronics, or they might short circuit in her presence. Hard for an engineer to comprehend, but if she can do things to my body from a distance of a thousand miles, she can probably do really amazing things from a few feet away, so why not?

The soil in the woods dried quickly, so I could move out there again. The mosquitoes must have had a crash breeding program going during the wet weekend, as they now were pest's as soon as the sun went down. Before the weekend, there had been hardly any.

I had scouted out a better location deeper into the woods, so I was farther away from the fumes from the apartments, and the path to the tent was a circuitous route around a couple of big downed trees. It was unlikely anyone would find it if going for a walk there. I did find somebody else's tent in there, but it was abandoned. Probably because of the rains.

When I slept in the tent, I connected myself to the ground, using a grounding rod outside the tent and a copper bracelet around my left ankle. I bought the cable from a nearby hardware store. Not a pleasant place to go, but I could do it for a short while by wearing my respirator. I managed to scare one of the cashiers with my mask.

I got the wire from the electrical department. There were many, many types of wire to choose from, and I could not seem to find a single-strand one, so I asked a staff member. He would not find me one from what I asked, but demanded to know what it was for. I was not going to tell him the truth, so I explained it was to ground a very sensitive piece of electronic equipment, using low voltages. He could only comprehend lightning rods, so I eventually had to go look for myself, after having wasted precious time in this toxic environment.

I did experiments shielding wires in various ways, measuring the improvements with my new gaussmeter. I found that I was more sensitive than this instrument, which could not show radiation below about 0.15 milliGauss (0.015 microTesla), which is what I measured by my tent in the woods, while it was 0.2 mGauss in my apartment during the day. In the evening, with my neighbors home, the lowest level in the apartment went up to 0.6 mGauss (0.06 microTesla).

When John moved out, I bought his old washer and dryer. I had been using only three sets of clothing that I kept washing in the bathtub, since my clothes got so contaminated at the laundromat. It took me weeks to get the washer cleaned for detergent residue, a type of chemical I am particularly reactive to. I hadn't used detergent for many years—first it was just to protect our waterways from this unnecessary pollution, later to protect myself against the toxic chemicals. Much more benign materials can be used, but there is less money in it for the corporate giants. And who can argue against incessant TV advertising? A case in point is that a best-selling brand was found inferior in an independent European study, and it still sells well there, due to TV advertising.

Dr. Q. arrived with more than a hundred treatment samples, which he muscle tested me for. Only the one vial marked "EPINEPHRINE" came up positive. Epinephrine is the clinical term for adrenaline. Years later, I was skin-tested for it, and had a weal, proof positive that I was allergic to it.

He added the "EPINEPHRINE" sample to the "EMF" and "brain" samples. When I picked them up, my hand quickly felt very warm, but it would be fine for the five to ten minutes the treatment would take.

I walked out the door with him, directly over to my tent in the woods. I had now named the place "Camp Secret," as only a few people knew about it, and only I knew exactly where it was. I had already stocked the tent with food and bottled water. No EMF sources within a hundred yards, not even a watch.

I kept a very low profile, not going farther than sixty feet away from my camouflaged tent, in case a neighbor would take a Sunday stroll in the woods. I did hear someone one evening but not near my tent. The weather was dry and the sun shone down through the trees, though it was not warm for June. One morning it was only 57° F (13° C), though it quickly warmed up to 67° F (19° C).

I had a lot of time to think, as there was nothing else to do. I could not read anything, and there was only so much to write in a letter. It occurred to me that people with this illness will always be pariahs and subjected to the unwitting whims of other people. It had taken decades just to control the cigarettes. Getting people to use less-toxic laundry products, fragrances and so on would be unrealistic in my lifetime. Even today, some smokers maintain there is no health risk. And would it be reasonable that a small minority of the population should deprive the rest of their choice for doing unhealthy things to themselves? There have been studies in California and Atlanta that suggested up to 15 percent of the population is bothered by these chemicals to some degree, though we "hard core" people are much fewer in numbers. Nobody knows how many we are, especially since many of us are never diagnosed and just wither away in painful mental stupors, especially among the less fortunate in society, who do not have the means to figure this out for themselves. With the epidemic of asthma among school children, there are sure to become more of us in the future, but hopefully society will be willing to face the problem beforehand. If nothing else, the fury of a mother with a sick child is something to behold, and perhaps stronger than the urge to smell as advertising tells us we must. And the need to have that perfect lawn. In Columbus, Ohio, home of the world's largest lawn care company, it is almost socially unacceptable to have a dandelion growing on the front lawn. The neighbors may complain that it affects their property value.

I thought about how amazing it was that a computer or a TV could affect me several feet away. But the radiation does reach further. In Europe, people have to pay a license fee to watch TV, and license-snoops patrol the neighborhoods with detectors that can pick up when a TV set is turned on inside a home. Spy agencies have long been able to pick up the radiation from computers, even through walls and from outside a building, to "read" what is on the screen. The military and other agencies use specially shielded computers, called TEMPEST, to avoid spies. The May 2009 issue of *Scientific American* had an article about this.

I stayed put until the food ran out after 42 hours. It was soon clear that the treatment had not helped. My initial truly amazing level of sensitivity had subsided a bit, but I knew that was only because I had not been exposed to EMF all that time. It would be unwise to push the envelope, though I did sleep on my balcony several nights when it was raining, and it was so cool the neighbors did not run their air conditioners right below the balcony. I was very lucky that my downstairs neighbor was away for weeks at a time during this spring. I seemed to have "made peace" with the refrigerator, so I could be in the apartment with it on, though I had to turn it off on the power strip every time I went in the kitchen.

I was still in contact with the healer in Dallas and kept a diary of when I could feel them work on me and what I observed. I was instructed to pause once in a while, relax and not think of anything, to make my mind more receptive to their transmissions (or whatever to call this). Usually, I could only sense a slight wave go through me, though once I suddenly felt drowsy and then suddenly very energetic.

Using the speakerphone, I kept in contact with the outside world and spent hours talking to my family and several other patients. In my little telephone support group, two fellow electrosensitives were especially helpful and cheerful, doing their best to keep my spirits up. The guy from Texas told stories of his experiences before he recovered. He now lives a fairly normal life, though his house is specially modified. When he was exposed to EMF, he used to lose muscle control in his legs and would be "flopping around like a dead chicken," as he described it. This would even happen if they drove under a high-tension power line. Being an engineer, he wanted to make sure that was really true, so he got his wife to drive around, with him blindfolded in the back seat. She would not give any hint when they crossed under one of those power lines, but he could tell every time. He sent me a copy of an article about him in the September 1994 issue of *Texas Monthly* magazine.

I was clearly not getting any better by staying in Columbus, and Debby told me I really needed to see her in person for her to work on me effectively. They were just doing "ambulance service" to keep me going. With the extraordinary demonstration she had given me of her special talent, how could I not go? In Dallas there is also more of an infrastructure to serve the many people there with this illness. The goodwill and volunteers I was relying on in Columbus would eventually run out, and winter in Ohio would be very bad.

But how to get to Dallas? Flying was out of the question. I looked long and hard at the shortest non-stop flight from Port Columbus to Dallas–Fort Worth airport. Two and a half hours in the air. A very long time if there is anybody with a laptop computer within fifteen or twenty feet — a virtual certainty. And many planes also had overhead television sets and even small display screens on the back of the seats. And once in there, there is no way to walk out. If five or ten minutes near my own laptop computer could produce such a profound effect, what would 150 minutes do?

Trains and Greyhound buses did not seem feasible either. There might be less electronic pollution, but there would be much more air pollution, as the people traveling by public transportation are the poorest segment of the population, the same most heavily targeted by corporations hawking toxic products such as fragrances and cigarettes. There are limits to how well my respirator works, and how long I could keep it on.

I told Debby of my dilemma. She confidently told me that I would find a way. "How can you be so sure?" I asked. She told me she knew because she could "see" me standing next to her in the future! She just didn't know how I would get there. If any other person on this Earth would have told me this, I would consider it rather out on the deep end, but her...

Then a colleague from work, Don, volunteered to drive me to Dallas in my own car, and then fly back to Ohio. He was busy with a project at work, so I had to wait six weeks, but now there was a way.

Life was getting more stable again, though complicated. It was a great relief not to have to try to keep my job going and at the same time also keep up my complex lifestyle, all while feeling as if having the flu.

I would run the exercise bike every morning on the balcony, while the sauna in the bedroom heated up. Being out there both kept the fumes from the bike's brake at bay, and I was away from the strong electromagnetic field around the sauna and the extension cord that ran from the kitchen to the bedroom.

Many afternoons, I could not use the balcony while one of the neighbors would dry their clothes because the exhaust fumes would drift up there. The two young women living next door were particularly bothersome, and they washed almost every day. A neighbor told me they worked every night at a restaurant, so it was probably work clothes.

While my own washer ran, I could not be inside, both because of the electromagnetic radiation from the motor in the washer and also because of the strong smell of chlorine from the water pouring into it. I would have to bring a chlorine filter for the machine with me back from Dallas, like the ones already on the kitchen faucet and my shower.

I would go for walks up to three times a day, mostly away from other people and traffic, but I also ventured across Dublin-Granville Road to a shopping mall. I found that the Big Bear supermarket there had a little bit of organic produce and a few other items.

While inside this Big Bear, I talked a little with a fireman who was shopping for the evening meal at his station. He was very nice and grasped my concern if I should have the need for ambulance transportation. He told me some of their crews used a lot of cologne and if that was a problem, they would give the patient an oxygen mask. When I told him that the oxygen mask itself would likely be bad too, he suggested I write a letter to the supervisors, explaining the situation. That would have to wait until my return.

When I walked up to the cashier, I got zapped by the refrigerated soft drink machine next to the checkout line. Then it seemed that the cash register itself was a problem — it contains a computer inside.

Dr. Q. had told me about someone else who was highly regarded for his work on the body's energy system. Dr. P. knew about environmental illness, though he had never seen one of "us" before. He clearly enjoyed the challenge and spent 45 minutes working on me. He put me on his table, after disconnecting the electricity to it. Then he muscle tested me for a large number of herbs to see if they were beneficial to me. Muscle testing is apparently standard fare in the world of alternative medicine. The idea is to ask the body questions, bypassing the conscious mind of the brain.

When I finally stood up, I had a clear sensation of something slowly floating through me, somewhat similar to the first treatments by Debby. I found that very encouraging. Perhaps I could still avoid going to Dallas.

At home, the armistice with the refrigerator was over. Again, it bothered me almost anywhere in the apartment, like it did when I had to abandon the apartment and move out in the tent. Since then, it had gone down to only bothering me when I was less than ten or fifteen feet from it. Dr. P. had cautioned me that temporary setbacks may happen while my body adjusted to his treatment. After a few hours, it simmered down again to be like it had been the day before.

I went to see him again two weeks later. I had not seen any remarkable improvement, but he was very optimistic. During one of the adjustments, my eyesight suddenly became completely clear for a few seconds. It was completely free of the disturbances and the haze that was always there, but then it went back again.

At home, all peace treaties were on hold with the refrigerator and the air conditioners outside. I had to make a hasty retreat to the tent in the woods. When I walked over the fields of the university farms, I could now feel the pulses from the electrical fences! Zap ... zap ... zap.... That had never happened before. It took almost two weeks to come back to the level of sensitivity as before the treatment, so I didn't dare do any more experiments. There was no way around going to Dallas.

One night when I was sleeping in the woods, a thunderstorm came rolling in. To be in close contact with the ground, I had been sleeping without the foam pad I normally use when camping. Now it turned out to be a problem, as I could feel when the lightning hit the ground, even when it seemed to be a few miles away. It was subtle and did not seem to pose a danger, but I stuck some clothing under me to get off the ground, and that worked.

Another night, a police helicopter kept circling overhead. Presumably, they were looking for some fugitive. I doubted anyone would stumble on my tent if running around in these woods, but maybe the helicopter would spot me with an infrared camera or night goggles. I kept still, and they may have thought I was a sleeping deer or such. Eventually, they moved away and I was not further disturbed.

It was really lucky these problems first got out of hand in the spring. It would not have been fun sleeping in the tent in the winter. We did get rain every few days, sometimes enough to make the ground soggy, so I dug a trench around the tent. I took the tent in to dry every few days and then slept the night on the balcony while it dried. I was concerned about getting the tent moldy so I could not be in it any more. It takes a long time to offgas a new tent, as they are full of plasticizers, flame retardants and pesticides to prevent mold growth. The year before, I had bought a new tent as a backup, which I aired out on the clothesline on many sunny days, but it was slow going.

Many nights in the woods, I could hear distant howling and yelping, which I took to be coyotes. The woods were bordered on two sides by large tracts of undeveloped lands. One night the coyotes sounded very close, but I never saw them.

The only animal encounter was when I woke up hearing something wandering near the tent, breaking twigs as it went. It was hard to guess how large it was, but it could not be larger than a coyote. It stopped right next to my tent, where I lay unmoving. When it had been standing there for a moment, I decided to break the ice by greeting it in a friendly voice. It instantly replied back with a very deep "HUNMPH?" I responded with a similar sound and shook the tent a bit to make it understand I was quite large. It uttered another HUNMPH sound and trundled away. Some days later, I went to put trash in our dumpster, where I encountered a rather annoyed raccoon that didn't appreciate my disturbance. It greeted me with another HUNMPH!

I continued my daily exercise-and-sauna detoxification program, which now took two hours every morning. I had briefly tried to do three sauna trips every day to speed things up, but Dr. Rea told me to step it down and not overdo it, during one of our telephone consultations.

In early July, my two friends who moved to the other end of town came and picked me up and drove me over to visit their new house. It was a beautiful sunny day, and they had taken great care to wear clothes free of laundry smells, so I could be near them. For a precious few hours, life felt normal, sitting in their backyard eating a pizza. It was the first pizza I'd had in a very long time. It agreed well with my stomach, showing that my food allergies were getting under control.

Their house was only 2½ years old and smelled strongly of formaldehyde. I didn't go inside, except for a brief tour wearing my mask. They had tried to make it comfortable for me by having all the windows open all morning, in the hope I could be inside. The house was so formaldehyde-laden I couldn't even be near one of the open windows on the outside!

For my two friends, this was a pretty ordinary day, while to me it was a brief return to a life of normalcy. A wonderful gift. I was only to experience one other day that year where sickness was not the 500-pound gorilla next to me.

Many years ago, I would listen to a morning radio program while eating breakfast. A disabled man in a wheelchair was the guest in the studio. He was asked what people should do when they encountered a disabled person. He simply responded that he would much prefer that people would just let him have a sense of normalcy. I remember thinking that was a very strange answer, but now I really understood.

A friend broke his leg the previous Christmas and needed help getting around for the next couple of months. He told me that experience made him realize how difficult it was to be disabled, and he became one of my greatest supporters.

For me, there was also something to learn here. Prior to becoming sick, I prided myself on my independence, that I could fully take care of myself in any way and didn't need anything from others. It was difficult having to ask other people for help, but that was a very positive experience as people really came through. The disappointment was the medical system, which one should expect to be helpful, but in many cases was quite the contrary.

It does not seem so surprising that I also became electrosensitive, since it was common among the severe patients in Dallas. I had certainly spent a lot of time in front of a computer screen. My first computer was a small mail-order machine I bought in 1981. It was quite primitive, with only 16 kilobytes of memory (in 2000, a typical desktop PC would have around 2000 times as much memory) and the processor ran at a meager one megahertz. It used my black-and-white television as the monitor.

Despite the shortcomings of that machine, and the ones I bought after it, I spent a lot of hours in front of the screen, especially when I later became a graduate student in computer engineering and made computers my livelihood.

Since I returned from Dallas, I substituted the computer for almost any type of paper. The computer was on from when I woke up and until bedtime, as it was essentially my desk. It is no wonder that it took a year to figure out that it was the cause of the burning sensations in my head, when it was always on. I had just assumed it was mold or air pollution.

It has later been suggested that the radar tower at the nearby airport, only a mile away, may also be a factor, as I must have been in the lower part of the area swept by this invisible finger. Or the new cell-tower only 200 yards away. Then there was the long-term exposure I was subjected to from the building transformer that was located right behind the wall in my office on the campus. It was only five or six feet away from my head. Perhaps that was a reason I had to give up the office the year before, as these burning sensations in my head would start after being there for only a few minutes, and my mind would simply not function clearly in there. It could hardly have been healthy to sit that close to a transformer stepping down thousands of volt to the regular 110 volt. A year later, I saw a French study (from *Archives of Environmental Health*, March 1998) that showed how workers exposed to a building transformer had lowered counts of white blood cells. My own count is low as well.

I continued to be in contact with Debby. She said I was easy to work with and asked me to continue with the journal I kept on what I observed of their remote work on me. She sometimes asked me to pay attention at a particular time, when her group of healers would work on me together. At those times I could often sense a lighter version of the "energy beam," and sometimes I would simply feel great with lots of energy for awhile.

I had been working on replacing the mercury amalgam fillings in my mouth over the last years. It is quite expensive to upgrade to a high grade of gold-platinum alloy, but the cheaper options include unhealthy metals such as nickel, which some people are allergic to, myself included. Metals seemed safer than plastic composite fillings. My dentist also refused to use them, as he didn't find them durable enough. I knew from my college classes in metallurgy that all metals corrode, it is only a question of how fast, so it does not seem like a healthy choice to use mercury in people's mouths, which is a highly corrosive environment.

Then I found a dentist who turned out to be such a delightful experience that I let him take the last three mercury fillings out of my mouth. His office was wonderful, though he would soon be moving to a new office with some carpeting. When I told him that less-toxic carpeting is available, he was sorry he hadn't heard that earlier, as the new carpeting was already ordered.

He talked me into using composite materials, instead of gold-platinum. It was a lot cheaper, allowing me to do all three now, and there is a concern about implanting any metals in the body of anyone who is electrically sensitive.

He scheduled me for a day when his dental hygienist wouldn't be there, so it would only be him and his assistant in the room.

The dentist was not familiar with electrosensitivity, but was quite open minded. The only problem was that his dental chair was quite "hot," but he moved it into position and disconnected it before I climbed in.

He tested me for which combination of dental material, bonding agent and anesticizer was best tolerated by my body, using the now-familiar muscle-testing. Some of the materials were clearly not welcomed by my body, but two composites were accepted, though not exactly loved.

With that decided, they took care of the first tooth, using precautions to minimize exposure to mercury fumes while the old filling was drilled out. They both wore respirators while I wore a special oxygen mask that only covered my nose. They also kept an oversize suction pipe trained on the work area, while a dental dam collected the debris so I would not swallow any of it.

A week later, he removed the last two fillings, from adjacent teeth. I had heard of other patients who saw dramatic improvements, including one very severe electrosensitive who got 90 percent better. I was not so lucky, though over the next couple of years I could see the mercury content in my blood go down to undetectable levels.

Some other patients had become very sick from the mercury removal process, but I was just extremely tired for three days, then back to normal.

It was very complex to organize the excursion, as I needed to line up volunteer drivers. It took me a full day to find the three people that it took to do the four rides. It sure is very cumbersome and time-consuming to be disabled.

I had done a lot of experiments on my car to see if I could reduce the electronic emissions. If I could just drive it for half an hour, that would make a tremendous difference. I tried shielding the emissions by wrapping steel around wires down in the foot well, even covering the entire foot well with a steel cage around my feet. The car itself was outfitted with a grounding wire which hung underneath and dragged on the road, like it is commonly done in Europe.

A colleague came up with the idea that ferrite cores may work, as they are used to reduce radio noise on quality cables for computer monitors.

All these changes did have some measurable effect. The highest radiation level was on the gas pedal, where it measured 35 milliGauss (3.5 microTesla) before I did any modifications. I was able to reduce it to about 25 milliGauss, but it didn't seem to make any difference. My feet would start burning as soon as I started the engine. I estimated I would need a 99 percent reduction, which was clearly not doable, so I gave up.

Two weeks before we left for Dallas, the floor tiles finally arrived. They had been sent by ship from the factory in France. A friend drove me up to the store in Marion, north of Columbus, and I shelled out $800 for 360 tiles. The plan was that a colleague would install them while I was in Dallas, so they had some time to offgas, but he would wait until we knew I would be able to return.

I have really been fortunate with all the people who volunteered to help during this very difficult period. It is in times of distress that one really sees the true face of humanity. While a couple people whom I thought I could count on turned their backs on me, many more stepped up and helped. There is hope for humanity.

11

Return to Dallas

I was very fortunate that my colleague, Don, volunteered to drive me down to Dallas. There was simply no other way to get there. He didn't want any payment for the effort and even offered to take the train home to save me money. What a guy! I insisted he take a plane back, of course.

It was my intention to stay in Dallas until I recovered enough to drive myself back home, however long that might take. I had loosely thought that it might take about three months. Three weeks before the departure date, it occurred to me that I might not be able to come back to Ohio again for a long time if no miracle was forthcoming in Dallas. I had heard stories of people who stayed down there for years. During my visit in the fall, I even talked with a woman from New England who was forced to pick a realtor from afar and mail off the key with instructions to sell the house and all her belongings.

The last three weeks before departure, I worked at going through my things and packing them up in crates, about a dozen in all. It was a big job to get through, and I didn't even do anything with the kitchen stuff. Lots of things were thrown out, and I went a dozen times to the Volunteers of America dumpster nearby, carrying bags full of clothes and other items. It was good to clean up, but I didn't want to do it too radically as I really expected to return in a few months.

I love books but couldn't read them at all. Still, I didn't want to part with more than a few of them. Some went to the VOA dumpster while others were given to friends or the library at my department. I tried to prune my collection of articles, but after getting very sick from handling them, that had to stop.

Some of the stuff I needed to send off by mail. The post office was three miles away from the apartment, and I managed to drive that far myself, though it was painful. I sat on the grass outside the post office for awhile to recover and wait for the lobby to be nearly empty of people. Then I walked in with the packages, wearing my respirator. Nobody batted an eye.

I could feel electromagnetic radiation when I walked near the counter, presumably from the computerized system they use. It took awhile for them to weigh in the packages, so I discreetly stepped away from the counter, but I could still feel it.

Outside the post office, I had to sit on the ground again for awhile, and again when I got home to ease the burning pain. This is really slow going. That was the only driving I did during those two months. I just had to try it, wishing for a miracle.

I had to venture in to the nearby Home Depot a couple of times to buy plastic crates for packing up my stuff. At least the smells didn't seem to hang so much in my clothes as fragrances do, so I could usually walk home without having to change the shirt. One time I must have been close to someone loaded with fragrances, as my shirt smelled so bad I had to walk home with my mask on. I was glad it was early morning, hoping nobody would wonder about a man carrying a box while wearing a big mask. That could perhaps create quite a stir, even before the terror attack on the Twin Towers in New York.

A week before departure, Don came to my apartment with a bag of clothes for me to wash in baking soda, so I was sure I could share airspace in the car with him. I also gave him a set of chemical-free deodorant, soap and shampoo to use.

I was concerned how long I could stand being in the car when we drove to Dallas. I seemed to do all right for the short trips I had been on during the last two months, when somebody drove, with me in the back seat, but what would it be like to drive several hours each day? I expected to need to stop once an hour to ground, but could I continue to do so through a whole day? Perhaps all that exposure could make me more sensitive, maybe even so much that we could not continue. We scheduled 4½ days for the trip, so there would be plenty of time for rest. If the trip could not be done in that amount of time, it could not be done. I planned on doing it in three days, then Don could use the extra time to see a couple of museums in Dallas, if he wanted to.

Wednesday, July 12, finally arrived, and I was ready. Two neighbors would keep an eye on the apartment, and my utilities had been scaled down to a minimum. The car was packed with camping equipment, my special foods and whatever else I would need for the trip and a lengthy stay. I even brought my answering machine and my laptop computer, in the hope of later using them — perhaps I could start working again from Dallas before returning to Ohio.

Don arrived at 1:00 P.M. He left his car at work, while another colleague,

Nancy, drove him to my apartment. She would later pick him up at the Port Columbus airport when he returned from the trip.

While Don went inside to change clothes, Nancy gave me two "get well" cards, signed by a lot of people —colleagues, managers, and customers. Very nice. I've signed a lot of those myself over the years; now it was my turn. Nancy uses scented products, so I could not be near her, but she took it well. She was one of the people who had taken turns to bring me groceries over the past two months.

Don came out again and locked the apartment. He now wore the clothes I had washed three times in baking soda and used the non-toxic toiletries I had supplied. Resolutely, he went in the driver's seat, while I jumped in the back, and we were off. Looking at the Columbus skyline as we circled around the city on Interstate 270, I wondered when I would see it again. My gut feeling was it would be quite awhile.

The trip started out well. I could feel the car's electronic emissions as a tingling sensation, but that was fine. As we got closer to Cincinnati, my feet started to feel warm, so we stopped at the rest area by the bridge over the Little Miami River. It would be awhile before the next rest area, and I'd rather not wait for the burning to start, as it was much harder to simmer down. I was delighted that I was doing so well, after driving a hundred miles.

Don drove us to a remote part of the rest area, and I spread out on the ground for about fifteen minutes. Don had never seen me do this before but was quite cool about it. I wondered what he really thought, though.

We continued through Cincinnati and followed I-71 towards Louisville, Kentucky. After an hour, my legs quickly went from feeling warm to burning. Don drove off the freeway, dropped me off next to a few trees and went to fill the gas tank. That way I could avoid the gasoline fumes at the gas station and do some much-needed grounding.

That evening we camped in a state recreational area in southernmost Indiana, close to the Ohio River. There was only one other tent in the entire campground, a great benefit of traveling on a weekday. They did have a campfire going, but we chose a campsite upwind so the smoke was not a problem.

It was very hot and humid there, and the sunset brought no relief. It was hard to fall asleep with the sweat constantly running down my face. Don slept in my new tent, which I had bought the year before and was still working on outgassing. I slept in my old tent that only smelled of plastic if it sat in the sun.

The next morning it was cooler, and fog had collected in the valley we were in. We didn't dawdle and were soon back on Interstate 64. So far, it had gone exactly as planned. I had chosen the route to be fairly direct, using freeways that had less truck traffic, so there were less diesel fumes to breathe. The small detour through Indiana gave us some choices on where to camp for the night.

The second day went smoothly, as we headed south through western Kentucky, through the northwest corner of Tennessee and in to Arkansas. We camped for the night at Village Creek State Park west of Memphis. This was the campground I couldn't find in the darkness on my way home from Dallas the previous November. It had more than a hundred campsites, and we had it all to ourselves. That is, we, the mosquitoes, the snakes, and the dense humid air. The excitement of the day happened when I nearly stepped on a good-size snake that was passing through our campsite around sunset.

Again, the day had gone according to my hopes and plans. In the morning I lasted two hours before we had to stop for me to rest and ground. In the afternoon, I would wear out faster, and the burnings would start sooner. We then had to stop once an hour. I didn't want to do it more often than that, and it went well.

The third day went well also, except I got bitten by some fire ants the first time we stopped in Texas.

Late in the afternoon, we arrived in Dallas. The rental office for Dr. Rea's condos was still open, and I got the key for room 222. Our roommate was Ted, a nice fellow. He used to be electrosensitive himself and had no problem not using the TV when I was around. Don had been very quiet on the entire trip but struck up a great conversation with Ted.

The apartment complex was right next to a big high-tension power line, which was probably what I could feel as soon as we arrived. Our apartment was a little further away from the power line than the front row of apartments, but not enough. I could feel it all the time, and my gaussmeter showed from 1.5 to 2 milliGauss everywhere in the apartment. It didn't help that our apartment was upstairs, so it was harder for me to ground.

The rental office closed soon after we arrived, and they had told me that all units were occupied anyway. I talked with some of the other residents, including two women who stayed in unit 122 right below us. It was better there, but not great. My gaussmeter showed about the same levels of radiation as upstairs, so being directly on the ground must be what made it better for me. The two women offered that I could stay the night on their living room floor.

I was also invited to try out an upstairs apartment farther away from the big power line, though there was also a smaller power line going down the street outside. It had a beautiful blue-tiled floor, but it felt the same as my own apartment.

I gratefully accepted the offer by the two women to sleep on the living room floor in apartment 122. The women were from New Jersey and North Carolina, respectively. Even when I slept on the floor all night, I could still feel the incessant tingling in my legs the next morning. The two women offered to switch apartments with Ted and me, but I needed to look for something better. I was already familiar with the Raintree apartments and knew they would probably not work for me, so I wanted to take a look at the EI trailer park in the southeastern suburb of Seagoville.

The woman from North Carolina was also interested in the place, so she went along. So did Ted — who had lived there for awhile in 1991 — just to see what it now looked like. I visited the place five or six times when I was in Dallas in the fall, so I was familiar with it already. One person I knew from then was still there. Several rooms were available.

We drove back to Dallas and discussed the options. The woman from North Carolina didn't like the place and did not want to move. She was leaning more towards giving up and moving back home, also because she was running out of money and hadn't seen much improvement from staying in Dallas and doing the treatment program. She did move back home again a few weeks later.

For me, there was a big concern about transportation. Food and bottled water can be delivered, but how to get the 26 miles to the clinic from Seagoville? Someone told me there was a guy who was an EI himself and made a living driving other patients around. His name was Lawrence (not his real name). We got hold of him, and he promised to drive me for $30 a day, round trip, with extra for shopping errands.

I moved that evening and chose to rent one side of a duplex. My room was about twelve feet (3.5m) on each side, with a tiny bathroom and a small covered porch in front. The entrance was a sliding glass door out to the porch, while two of the walls were dominated by large windows. All surfaces, including floor and ceiling, were covered by steel plates coated with a ceramic surface that was similar to old refrigerators, but in a cheery yellow that would not have made it into any kitchen.

Don spent the night in a tent on the lawn outside my window. It was cooler than inside, so he preferred it that way.

The next afternoon, the thermometer reached 111 degrees F (44°C) on my porch. Don drove off to the enclosed mall in nearby Mesquite to cool off, while I braved the heat at my new home. An enclosed mall did not sound like a place I could be, and I might as well get used to living in this heat anyway. My room had a window air conditioner, but the electromagnetic radiation would have been murder on me.

Late in the afternoon, we drove in to Seagoville to visit Dolores's house. She once lived at the camp for six years, until she got this house. To help pay for the mortgage, she rents out three bedrooms to other EIs. I wanted to make contact there to see if there was a possibility to share rides to the clinic. There were currently two renters, one of whom I met in the fall, but neither of them went to Dallas regularly. Still, it was nice to see a familiar face.

Don's plane left early the next morning. I had arranged with Lawrence to drive both of us to Dallas, drop Don off at the airport and then deliver me to Dr. Rea's clinic. I later learned that Lawrence had slept in his car in Dolores's driveway to make sure we made it to the airport in time for Don's very early plane.

12

The Seagoville Camp

The camp was started more than twenty years ago by Ray Scott, who owned a piece of land outside Seagoville. One day Dr. Rea asked him if a homeless environmental patient could park his trailer on Scott's land, and that was the start of it. Over the years, more and more has been added to the camp, which also has moved two times. Initially, it was just a collection of camping trailers that had been modified. Some steel buildings were also built on skids, so they could be transported.

At its present location, the camp consists of more than two dozen structures, most of them stationary. They are arranged in a rough circle around a center lawn, which originally housed some long-gone travel trailers. Most of the old travel trailers eventually became moldy and unusable and were removed.

In its heyday in the early 1990s, the camp held around two dozen residents—some people even say there were thirty. Today, there is room for fourteen, though when I moved in, there were only seven renters, plus the owners. The kitchen is shared among the renters; it is hard to imagine it being used by twenty to thirty people!

There are forty-seven acres of land, most of it lakes. Since the land was picked over by bulldozers for gravel mining decades ago, nature had reclaimed it with plenty of bushes and trees, while there is a thriving ecosystem with large fish and turtles in the lakes. The camp itself only takes up a few acres on the southern side of the property, while the rest of the land is left wild as a buffer zone towards the neighbors. On two sides, there were two operating gravel pits. The third side, to the south, is uninhabited forest and swampland. Only on one side are there houses, with the nearest two hundred yards from the camp.

Ray Scott lived in the camp himself, together with his wife, until a house was built for them at the other end of the property. It was built of safer materials and placed on fourteen-foot-high stilts, like the type used in flood-prone areas of southern Louisiana. The purpose of raising the house was to get above the mold, which tends to be worst closer to the ground. This method was not very successful.

Mrs. Scott died in a car accident, and a few years later, Ray Scott died himself. On his deathbed, he gave the property to his live-in managers, Ellie and Jock (not their real names), on the condition the place was carried on to help future EIs in need.

Jock was about 85 years old, a veteran of World War II. He was a blue-collar worker from Ohio who moved south to Louisiana when he married Ellie, who taught French at a college. When Ellie got sick with environmental illness, they moved to Dallas to be near the doctors there.

Jock had worked a lot with asbestos and was eventually diagnosed with asbestosis, another illness that industry delayed acceptance of for a long time. He never received his just compensation for this illness that was a daily problem for him, along with other problems.

Ellie and Jock lived in the camp themselves but had their own private kitchen in a little shack of black painted steel. At the previous location of the camp, this shack had been the laundry room. It was about twenty feet long, with a later addition at the end, that was a small low-ceilinged living room for them. It was very rustic, only the living room part had any insulation, while the kitchen section had just one layer of thin steel walls to the outside.

The rest of us shared a much larger kitchen shack, which was a simple wood frame building covered with corrugated steel on both the roof and the walls, and a slab of raw concrete as floor. There was no insulation at all, so it was very hot in the summer and very cold in the winter. It has since been insulated.

The kitchen shack was sixty feet long and about thirty wide, divided into four rooms. One room was the kitchen; one held six washers and six dryers. The remaining two rooms each held a row of refrigerators, one for each resident, and some spares.

Behind the kitchen was an open patio, next to a pond. A very nice setting, as we could sit and watch turtles swim in the water and big white birds wade along the shore on their tall legs spearing frogs with their long beaks.

The whole camp had a post-apocalyptic feeling to it, like something out of an old Mad Max movie. It really looked like what it was: a refugee camp. We were exiles from the toxic world outside and were not really free to leave, as there were few other places to go. But to me, it was a good place that summer, as it finally seemed I had found a place I could live in peace and could start working on recovering.

To limit the fumes from the vehicles, the camp was set back about two hundred yards from the road. The driveway ended in a parking lot, from where one had to walk in to the grassy campus. The kitchen shack was about 250 feet from the loading zone and further from the parked cars.

The building nearest to the parking lot was a strange contraption. It had five rooms strung around three sides of the building. Three of the rooms faced the loading zone. One was the biggest room on campus, designed for two people, but I once saw four sleep in there. The middle room was aptly named "the tunnel," as it was deep, narrow and windowless, except for the glass door. It was now used to store electrical space heaters, probably because nobody wanted to live there. The third room was the nicest on campus. It was spacious with a tiled floor and large windows. In camp lingo, each separate room was called a unit.

Around the corner was a small room, and in the back was a tiny room that was made from a small camping trailer that was cut open and grafted to the side of the building. This one had a tiled floor, while three of the others had floors covered with the too-cheery yellow porcelainized steel.

The transformer for the whole campus hung on a pole next to the building, and right in front of it was a big breaker panel with the electrical meters. This made the building unusable for most people with severe electrical sensitivities. In the entire time I lived there, I was only inside it twice during power outages.

On the "low EMF" side of the campus was a row of trailers and a couple of buildings. One building was a small house that was already on the land before it became the camp. It was a regular stick-built house with stucco walls on the outside and wooden floors. It had been completely gutted on the inside and made into two separate units, each with its own bathroom. The floor, walls, and ceiling were the yellow porcelainized steel plates. The door to the bathrooms was a cotton curtain, as it was in almost all the units.

Next door was an old aluminum mobile home from the 1950s. It was about forty feet long and twelve wide, with two rooms and a bathroom. Again, all covered in the yellow porcelain. It had a nice covered porch in the front and a great view to the lake in the back.

Then came a moveable home on skids, that had been custom built from the start to house environmentally sick people. It was built by Dr. Lattieri, a dentist who built several such moveable homes and trailers. It was constructed of heavy steel plates and must be very difficult to move. It had a bedroom, living room/kitchen and a bathroom, all in a package thirty feet long and perhaps twelve wide. The bathroom had a separate outside door, which some residents have used as an airlock instead of using the regular front door. One resident went one step further and always took a shower and changed her clothes before going in to ensure a pristine environment inside.

Farther on, in our tour of the row, were a couple of aluminum travel trailers that had most of their interiors removed and then all surfaces were covered with aluminum tape.

Then came a small moveable building, another Lattieri design, I believe. I found this one to be most depressing. It was a claustrophobic little cell, no more than twelve feet on each side, with two tiny windows and steel walls in a mind-numbing dark blue color.

Behind it was a building made entirely of the golden yellow porcelain steel plates, both on the inside and on the outside. Surprisingly, there was very little rust, though I doubt it would work in the wetter northern states. It was an odd-looking duplex, with a room at each end and a shared bathroom in the middle. Sharing the bathroom between two renters produced so many conflicts that now the building is only rented out as a whole unit. It was a good choice for a couple living together or a patient with a caretaker. The rooms had very large windows, making them look like a fishbowl. A covered front porch rounded off this unusual structure.

The row of units ended with the recreation room. It was a 30-foot-long one-room building, made of corrugated steel on the outside, with a raw concrete floor and the porcelainized steel on the walls and ceiling. A big covered porch ran along the whole front side, where the only public pay phone was located. The building had for several years been rented to a woman who had been extremely electrosensitive, though she no longer was. It had been the only unit that would work for her. There was no bathroom in the building, so she had to use the shared bathroom in a little hut next to the kitchen.

While she was extremely electrosensitive, she could not be in her building most of the time during the summer because of the air conditioners on the other nearby units. She had to build a screened-in room well away from the main camp, behind a small hill. The room was about ten feet long and six wide, with an overhanging steel roof. The walls were framed of steel rods with aluminum mosquito netting. The floor was stacked concrete blocks on a raised foundation of dirt. Very rustic, but a heaven when you need it. She called it her Oasis, though most people referred to it as The Cage.

My own unit was a part of a duplex and stood where the levels of EMF were the lowest in the main campus area. It was near the kitchen shack and sixty to eighty feet away from the other units, except my neighbor in the other side of the duplex. My neighbor was also highly electrosensitive, so we simply kept the breakers off for the whole building most of the time. The exception was when he wanted to run a fan in his room at night before going to bed. When it was on, we both had to be out of our rooms.

The camp was set up so we could arrive with just our clothes on our backs, and some people came close to that. It was not uncommon to arrive, expecting to stay for a couple of weeks, and end up staying a year.

The kitchen was fully equipped with pots and pans, and each person was issued a refrigerator, a set of plates, utensils and a private shelf in the kitchen.

Each of our units had a metal hospital bed, which was covered with seven mattress pads of organic cotton and two cotton blankets. Mattresses were not used, as it takes a lot of time to offgas their flame retardants and other nasties. There are organic chemical-free mattresses, but they are very expensive and many people have problems with the smell of untreated cotton. Also, they cannot be washed, so it would not take long before they would become smelly with the chemicals that some of us sweat out, now that the body finally is given a rest from the daily onslaught. The mattress pads were easy to wash and worked well, though not as soft as a real mattress.

It was best to keep the room as free of stuff as possible. Many of us stored our belongings outside. I had a nice covered front porch with a little steel cabinet on it. It used to be a hospital nightstand. Eventually, I acquired two steel trash cans and several big plastic buckets to store my things in.

Each unit had a window air conditioner and a small television. The TV set was placed in a little metal cabinet which hung on the outside wall. The screen could be seen through a glass window in the wall. That way the fumes from the hot electronics were not a problem, and exited the metal box through a small chimney to the outside.

I could not use either the TV or the air conditioner, because of the radiation. Fortunately, my room had stucco walls on the outside, which did not make it quite as hot as those with all-metal walls. Some folks would turn on their air conditioners to cool down their units in the evening, and just stay at a safe distance while it was running.

Electromagnetic sensitivity was not much of an issue at the Environmental Health Center in the early 1990s, and little was known about it, so no special precautions were taken in the construction of the camp, which Dr. Rea was involved in as a consultant.

As I would slowly realize, metal buildings are a great choice for less toxic construction, but not always for electrosensitives. The metal blocks and reflects electromagnetic radiation, which means that radiation from any source inside the building would bounce around inside, instead of simply passing through the nearest wall. I got a lesson on that one evening when I was having a conversation on my speakerphone. I was getting attacked by the mosquitoes outside, so I went inside my room, leaving the speakerphone on its pedestal outside the door. I continued the conversation through the screen door, but as soon as I went inside, the phone bothered me. If I went outside, it subsided again.

The metal floor made it harder to ground myself, apparently because the metal blocked the flow of energy from my body down to the ground. If I walked barefoot on the metal, I could feel an electrical tingle in my feet. I was fine wearing shoes or when on the bed, raised above the floor, as long as I was not "loaded" with a charge I needed to release. Then I definitely felt better outside. Otherwise, I felt good inside — much better than in Ohio, and anywhere else.

The room had big windows on three of the walls, which really helped. I first realized how much the big windows helped when I entered other units with small windows, and would feel electrical tingling in my body, even though there was no other source than myself. So my choice of unit to stay in was the best; I just didn't know it until much later. I just went with my gut feeling and a sense that being away from most of the neighbors was a good thing.

Years later, I tried several steel buildings, which did not have a steel floor, and did well in them. Eventually I had one built myself.

In the heyday of the camp, in the early 1990s, the overcrowding got the inmates to nickname the place Stalag 17. Others made up a T-shirt with the name "The Last Resort" on it, with some trailers drawn underneath. It is good to see that humor never dies.

Some of the neighbors along the road were said to believe that the camp is some kind of resort, as the place looks rather idyllic from the outside, with its lakes and lush surroundings. On summer weekends, we would often see a few vehicles coming up our driveway, just to take a look, and some would trespass, trying to fish in the lakes.

There was always the concern that a truckload of drunk teenagers would come roaming in on a Friday night and douse us with fragrances or pesticides.

The good thing about living in this neighborhood was that people were not compelled to have that perfect lawn and apply copious amounts of pesticide in order to rid it of that nefarious invader: the mighty dandelion.

13

Fellow Refugees

Most of the residents in the camp were not very social. The only person I really could talk to was Sue (not her real name), who had been living there for about a year when I arrived. I knew her a little from my trip to Dallas the previous year and was glad for the company. We spent many afternoons under the big pecan tree, while looking at the wildlife in the pond behind the kitchen shack.

She was the resident "pesticide queen," as she was amazingly sensitive to this type of poison. It would take so little to set her off, that I was a bit skeptical at first. She fully convinced me the day I came back from Dallas, and at a distance of thirty feet, she asked me where I had been, as she could smell pesticides on me! She had never said that before. On the way back from Dallas, I needed to get a film developed, and Lawrence had taken me to a Wal-Mart store. Their photo shop was right inside the door, so I was only in the building for two minutes. It was not so different from the children that are so sensitive to peanuts, that manufacturers of candy bars now label their products with a warning if their product is made in a facility that also processes peanuts. With a shower and a change of clothes, I was cleansed of the incident, and Sue could be around me again.

With that level of sensitivity, Sue was more concerned about the pesticide contamination of our foods than anyone else. The problem is that even if the food is organically grown, it can become contaminated between the farm and the dinner table in a variety of ways. If the store sprays for bugs while the produce is on the shelf, it may receive some of the fallout. While most stores in Dallas spray on a regular schedule, Whole Foods only sprays when insects have been observed, but they still spray.

Then there are the stories about truckers who spray their load of organic produce to ensure there will not be any insects found when the load arrives at the destination. Apparently, the trucker has some financial interest in the insect-free produce, and none in the food being free of poison.

To protect herself, Sue basically only ate foods from two sources: Her meat came from an organic farmer in Iowa, who shipped it directly to her. Her vegetables came frozen from the farm. She bought her frozen vegetables at a smaller health food store called Roy's, which never sprays. They use baited traps, if needed.

Every couple of weeks, a nurse would come to the camp to give her intravenous vitamins and minerals. It was the same nurse every time, from some home health-care agency. She stunk strongly of laundry products, so I had to flee every time she showed up. Poor Sue could not run. Sometimes I would get a whiff of the nurse, and my sinuses would burn for the rest of the day, and it also affected my brain. Sue asked the nurse several times if she could wash her clothes in something less toxic, at least just try washing them in baking soda, but it was just too much effort.

Sue bought a car during the fall and finally started to go out in the world a little again. I escorted her on her first trip to Dr. Rea's clinic in many months, and she did fairly well there, though she could detect faint amounts of pesticide. That was probably from the other patients' clothes and what had been tracked in on shoes.

Another resident was a woman who had arrived a month before me and went home late in the fall. She had been exposed to a lot of pesticides, which are used extensively in the farming area she came from. Apparently, she had so much of it in her body that Sue could not be anywhere near her or her unit. It was simply coming out of her, now that her body had the opportunity.

My neighbor in the other half of the duplex was rarely outside the camp. He was so sensitive that he could not be in his room or any other building during the day. He didn't really know what bothered him in his room but thought it could be the insulation material in the walls, as it was worst when it was hot.

In an attempt to cool down his room at night and rid it of whatever was bothering him, he would set up a big fan in the evening. We had negotiated that he would turn it off at 9 P.M., so I could go to bed. Since I only had a flashlight, I followed the sun, and rose by first light.

As the summer progressed and it became darker earlier, we would have hordes of mosquitoes coming out of the ponds once the sun went down. The only way for me to avoid their bites was to keep walking, as there was no other place for me to go inside. As it got cooler late in the fall, the need for walking around the last hours before I could go inside my room continued, but instead of giving the mosquitoes a moving target, it was to stay warm. I wore off a lot of shoe leather on those concrete walkways.

Living this closely with a group of people is always a challenge. I did it for almost four years while in college, where I lived in a student co-op. Then, most of us attended the same engineering school and tended to have other things in common. In Seagoville, we were a group of dissimilar people, who had been thrown together by this illness, not by any desire for communal living. Although there were few philosophical conflicts—very few supported the Republicans, for instance — there were many other causes for conflict. Everybody had their special needs, which sometimes conflicted with other people's needs, like my neighbor's nightly fanning of his room. Still, we had a sense of camaraderie, borne out of the reality that we were all in the same boat in stormy waters.

During my first summer there, we were only five people who used the shared kitchen, and even when we later were more fully occupied, there were never more than ten kitchen users.

One person had been living in the camp for a number of years. During a period with few residents, she only shared the kitchen with one other person. She had then developed a sense of propriety and seemed to consider fully half of the kitchen as "her territory," which was clearly marked by personal items left on the table and the counters. She would also leave various items to be stored or offgassed on our common patio, instead of more appropriately behind her own unit or behind the cook shack.

Another problem was with a highly electrosensitive person, like myself. Neither of us could walk in to the washing machines, if any of them were running, as the radiation from the motor would give us the pains. He had also a problem making clothes work for him and was constantly washing the same pieces over and over again, all day long. For me to do my laundry, I had to wait until his machine stopped, so I could go in and start mine. But then he had to wait for mine to stop, before he could start his.

The logical solution would be that we started our machines at the same time, but somehow that didn't really work either. For awhile, I washed as soon as I got up in the morning, but eventually I moved to another set of washing days. We were allowed to wash either Monday-Wednesday-Friday or Tuesday-Thursday-Saturday. Nobody washed Sunday, which was a welcome respite from the eternal drone of the machines.

During my first Dallas trip the previous fall, I had met a woman from China. She had become ill after her office was remodeled with new carpeting and other things.

During her stay in Dallas, he electrosensitivity surfaced, so she no longer could stay in Dr. Rea's apartments and moved to the camp in Seagoville. When her visa ran out, she flew home with the intent of raising more money and then coming back in May.

One of the EIs kept in regular contact with her by phone, but suddenly lost all contact in May. Her situation had been deteriorating rapidly. She lived in an apartment on the top floor of a tall building, which had a lot of radio transmission equipment on the roof. Soon she was too sick to even fly out of there and was in constant excruciating pain. She then decided on the only way out and took her own life. I had heard about other suicides among EI patients, but this was the first by a person I knew.

A memorial service was held in October at the library in the clinic. About a dozen people attended the beautiful ceremony, which was accompanied by soft music and the reading of oriental poems. It was recorded and pictures were taken, which were all sent to her family in China.

Most lives claimed by this illness seem to be from suicides, while the illness itself kills more indirectly through organ failures or anaphylactic shock. The previous year, a patient from Germany was living at the camp. He died because his rib cage collapsed. The doctors in Germany had given him massive doses of steroids, which had made his bones very brittle. He died in the hospital.

The next suicide happened at Christmas. A former camp mate, whom I also knew from my visit in the fall, had become too impoverished to stay there and had moved back where he originally came from. A friend allowed him to live in a garden shed, under very primitive conditions. He did poorly there, and his health deteriorated. He had once become allergic to all foods and had to be fed intravenously, and he had recovered his ability to eat. Now his difficult living conditions apparently were causing him to become resensitized to his food, and he didn't wish to start over again — nor did he have any money for the medical bills — so on Christmas Day, he committed suicide. More would follow.

14

Energy Work

My top reason for coming back to Dallas was to see Debby, this amazing person, who from a distance of a thousand miles could bring me out of the terrible situation I was in, that evening in May. I would probably have come anyway, as Dr. Rea would be my only other hope, and staying in the tent in Ohio was not a long-term solution.

It was with great expectations and curiosity that I showed up for the first appointment. I was received by her and the two apprentices, who had also worked on me remotely. I wasn't sure what to expect but was relieved that Debby didn't look unusual at all. No flowing robe, bare feet, strange hairstyle, mysterious makeup or gaudy jewelry. Instead, she was a radiant lady around fifty, with blond hair and wearing a simple suit. She could easily have been any sort of business manager.

We did a little small-talk, and then she asked me to lie down on the massage table. She said that metal objects would interfere with their work, so I would have to remove my belt, glasses, wallet, pocket knife, etc. Wait a minute! How did she know I carried a pocket knife? She just smiled her little smile, that I would get to see many times.

The two apprentices then took turns to "scan" my body, by moving their hands over me, starting at my head. Then they talked a little about what they had sensed. Apparently, Debby can "see" the status of my body directly, as she didn't do the scanning with her hands. She asked about the bones I broke in my leg when I was 13 and about a minor injury on my right ankle, which at first I couldn't remember. Very impressive.

Then they started balancing my body's "energy system," the same system that oriental doctors talk about. In China they refer to this energy as "chi," while "subtle energy" is used more in North America.

I was told that my extreme sensitivity to EMF was caused by the blockages of these energy pathways. I had heard about these things before and had seen the meridians drawn on pictures of the human body but was not real clear on how it works. But then, how many people understand how a little pill can knock out an infection? And some of the drugs that are prescribed by physicians are not really understood as to how they work, even by the pharmaceutical companies.

The apprentices did most of the work, while Debby supervised. Each session usually started with one apprentice sitting down by my feet and touching certain spots on the bottom of my feet with her fingers. This drains the excess energy stored in my body — out through her hands, through her body and down to her feet and into the ground.

I am a human battery, accumulating the electrical energy I receive when exposed to electromagnetic radiation. A person with a normal healthy body simply lets the energy pass through without even knowing it.

Being an engineer, I can understand how pulsed magnetic fields can induce an electrical current in a conductor, such as the human body. The same principle is used to generate electricity in both big power plants and in a car's alternator. It just never occurred to me that live bodies do it too.

While I was being "grounded," another apprentice usually put her hands on other parts of my body, such as the back of my neck and on my chest, apparently to release stuck energy, which then moves down to the other apprentice's hands. Debby would then sometimes join in and do some healing work by sending "white light" into a specific part that she decided to work on, such as my head or stomach.

Their treatment was so relaxing that I often forgot to breathe, which they would remind me to do! Besides the obvious need to breathe, the action of breathing is also essential for moving the energy around. It moves upwards when I breathe in, and downwards when I breathe out.

Eventually, I was able to feel this movement of energy myself. After just a few treatments, I could already feel the draining of my excess energy as a light tingle in my lower legs— a much more pleasant feeling than the rough vibration and burning sensation when I get "loaded up" with energy from exposures to EMF.

To have a better connection with the ground, they all took their shoes off before working on me. To improve my own natural release of energy, they suggested I go barefoot as much as possible and to get shoes with leather soles. Going barefoot at the camp proved to be difficult, as there were a lot of burrs in the grass. The concrete walkways would get so hot in the afternoon sun that I could not walk on them either. Broken glass was also a problem.

I had been instructed to lie on the ground several times a day to drain excess energy that way, or do it by holding onto a tree. I had already started doing that before I left Ohio and continued to do so. I was particularly fond of a young tree in front of the Environmental Health Center, where I really could feel the energy run out through my hands. Sometimes it would run so strongly that my hand felt warm. After three to ten minutes, the sensation would stop, so I knew when I was "grounded" as well as I could be on my own. Bigger trees with thick bark didn't seem to work as well.

A lot of unusual things are seen at Dr. Rea's clinic, so people didn't take much notice of someone holding onto a tree in the front yard. I was hardly the first to do this anyway, though a few patients took pictures of me doing it.

I found that it worked best if I took my shoes off and mentally focused on my feet and the hands on the tree. Mind and matter are surely connected. There also seems to be a sort of "conduit" between the hands, so I can move this energy from my right hand, through the arms and out the left hand. This I could use to drain excess energy from my head. I'm very much a "head person," which apparently causes accumulations of energy in my head. By placing the right-hand fingers in the middle of my forehead and holding onto a tree with the left hand, I could drain excess energy off that way. It was mostly then that the hands felt warm, like an electrical cord with too much current running through it.

I can redirect energy by breathing out, and focus my mind on where to send it. I once tried with my nose, and it did feel warm doing that!

When I sat up on the massage table after the first few sessions, I would feel dizzy, and one of them would escort me out to ground with a tree. Within a few minutes, the world would steady itself again. I was told the dizziness is caused by the delay in getting all parts of the body to arrive at the new equilibrium.

After these sessions, I would feel relaxed and usually pretty good. Sometimes my vision would also be completely crisp, which was otherwise rare. Unfortunately, this bliss didn't last long. No more than 2 to 3 hours, and sometimes I would run into a perfumed person or a cell phone right outside, and the effect would be gone.

I went twice a week for these sessions with Debby and her "energy workers," as we patients dubbed them. It was mostly the same three people, but others joined from time to time. Sometimes five women worked on me at the same time. They often joked about how I must enjoy having all these women all over me. Being the only male patient at the time, I just had to grin and bear it. Debby said they did have a few male apprentices, but they didn't have time during the week. They should also be more serious types. The group here certainly kept things upbeat.

After they'd worked on me for a month, the whole group put their hands on my torso, and Debby instructed them to send me loving energy. At the same time, I should focus on the feelings for a person I've once loved romantically. Debby would quickly wise-crack: "Not THAT kind of thoughts!" My thoughts were pure. I had already learned that they can read emotions very clearly.

This treatment was done to open up the energy from my heart, the heart chakra, which was completely blocked and had been for years. At an earlier session, they had all put their hands on my heart and connected to my heart energy. They could feel old sadness stored there, which had been suppressed for many years. Some of them had tears in their eyes!

Now I was to be connected with my higher emotional center, the heart chakra. I felt a warmth in my chest while we were doing this, a sensation that gradually would become commonplace for me.

When I later redid the exercise on my own, it felt like the floor disappeared and I was falling into a deep dark well. Fast. Faster than a free fall. My reflexes immediately pulled the brakes, closing the connection to my heart center. I tried a dozen times, and it was the same each time. I could only endure this sensation of accelerated fall for a few seconds at a time.

At the next appointment, Debby explained that it was old stored emotions that I was releasing. She suggested I talk to Dr. Cole, a psychotherapist who also volunteers as an "energy worker." With Dr. Cole, I was able to identify the sensation as simply raw fear. She also encouraged me to continue releasing it, in small pieces at a time.

Every time I tried, the frightening sensation of speeding down a dark hole would happen immediately, which I could only stand for a few seconds, no matter how much I steeled myself. I am not particularly scared of heights, but this was something else. I could now easily start it at any time. If that was what it took, so be it, and I kept it up, a few dark seconds at a time.

For about a week, this process was so close to me, that I had to mentally "hold my hand on the brake" all the time, instead of having to trigger it intentionally. It would come up every time I would relax and work on releasing excess energy. Then it slowly subsided, first by only happening when I intended it to. I was also able to endure it longer.

At the end of a session, Debby asked me to stay and rest on the massage table a bit. She must have motioned the others to leave, because we were suddenly alone. Feeling "up for it," I mentally "loosened the brake" and this time I had the pleasant sensation of peacefully descending, instead of the brutal fall. Debby came up and stood next to me, smiling her silent encouragement.

Soon afterwards, the sensation faded away completely. The process had lasted about a month. Debby explained that she could probably have released it for me in one go, but then I would have been so distraught that I would have been unable to care for myself and would have had to be institutionalized for a while. I believe it!

Much later, I would hear about another therapy that could also do this. Called Rolfing, it is a sort of brutal massage that mechanically releases stored emotions in the body — memory and emotions are stored throughout the body, not just in the brain. I've never tried Rolfing myself.

A month into the treatment, I tried to drive my car for the first time since I left Ohio. I needed to gauge my progress and see how much longer before I could drive home again. First I drove over to Dolores's house in Seagoville. It was seven minutes away, and went well, with just some tingling in my feet.

Then I got overconfident and drove a detour home, about a fifteen-minute drive. That was clearly too much. My feet burned uncontrollably and for the next couple of days, my sensitivities were much worse. After that, I didn't drive it for a month and then only every couple of weeks to either Dolores's house or the five miles to Seagoville, with a stop halfway for grounding. One of the neighbors at the camp hadn't been able to drive her car for two years. I hoped I would recover much sooner than that.

I also tried to fire up my laptop computer for the first time in three months. I had brought it in the hope I could start working remotely from Texas, before going home to Ohio. Alas, I didn't last five minutes in front of the computer, even though it has a low-radiation LCD flat screen and I used a separate keyboard and mouse to keep a little distance. This recovery was clearly going to take some time.

I had told my father about what was going on with these treatments, and he showed great interest, which I mentioned to Debby. She asked if he would be willing to let them work on him remotely, as an experiment. He agreed. Debby tried but could not get through. She asked me to coach my dad to relax and "let them in." I did so when I talked with him on a Sunday in the middle of August. He tried while we were talking and immediately felt a warmth and tingling in his arms and hands, which was similar to what I had experienced a few months before in Ohio. He was seven time zones away, and still it worked! I recorded the time at 11 A.M., my time.

At my next appointment with Debby, two days later, she volunteered that she had suddenly gotten through to my dad Sunday morning around 11 A.M. I had not said anything at all about it.

One day Debby was on a trip to Arizona; the session was conducted by her most experienced apprentice. They apparently felt like doing something special, so one of them put her hands on my chest and leaned heavily. She asked me to breathe in and feel the heaviness of her hands, to lift them up with my lungs. We did that a few times. Then she asked me to press against her hands with my mind! I had to experiment several times and got feedback from her when she could sense that I was getting closer. Then suddenly, her hands felt like a feather touch, and I could breathe unrestricted, while she obviously exerted herself pressing her hands down on my chest. Amazing!

I figure George Lucas must have understood these things when he created the *Star Wars* movies. "Use the Force, Luke" suddenly doesn't seem so farfetched.

Encouraged by these experiments, I tried to help my neighbor Sue a few weeks later. She was having a minor health crisis and felt crummy. I now understood that sending other people healing thoughts can indeed be helpful. No wonder churches have prayer sessions for people in crisis. So I tried to think of Sue's well-being intensely, like when we did the experiment with the hands on my chest. Sue said she felt some sudden warmth in her chest, but at the same time I suddenly felt really drained. Debby later explained that I had probably given away some of my own life force, which is not the way to do this. I don't have enough life force as it is, so I shouldn't play around with these things. Healers have to be healthy to work on other people.

Another day, when the apprentice started draining excess energy through my feet, she couldn't get it going. It turned out she wasn't doing it right. Debby said she otherwise had a procedure called "roto rooter" where she momentarily reverses all energy flows in the body, to get things flowing. I did try this a year later, and it didn't seem so dramatic. This time, however, Debby proceeded to do something, which got me to fly off the table as if a big hand suddenly lifted me up. She was satisfied with this response, though I was then so dizzy I was escorted out to hug a tree afterwards.

I have always been a "head person," constantly interested in learning new things, which was obviously a very good thing in a career consulting on the ever-changing world of computers. It also made it harder to calm down my thoughts, as new ideas and thoughts would constantly bubble up to fill the void. For that reason, I always had paper and pen ready next to my bed, as many good ideas would come to me while falling asleep at night.

Perhaps this focus on just "living in my head" was a reason most of my symptoms were concentrated there, from the ever-tender sinuses, to the blurry vision and the "foggy" mind, as well as the occasional numbness of the facial skin and the numerous pains that would show up in response to exposures. Most of the symptoms only happened in the right side of the head, an indicator that the system was severely out of balance.

Debby encouraged me to try meditation. I was instructed to simply lie down, close my eyes and try to calm my mind. Calming my mind was the hard part.

My meditation sessions were usually an almost sleeplike relaxation, which seemed like a good thing. One afternoon in the sweltering heat of a Texas August, I could suddenly sense the pulse in my chest. It was very strong, though still running at a peaceful rate. My eyeballs suddenly turned around in their sockets, behind my closed lids, and I felt like I was slowly descending in an elevator. I saw a lot of bluish light, as if I were looking at a clear blue sky. Then a pulsing sensation slowly moved all over my head, front and back, up and down. I opened my eyes, wondering if an outside light source created this blue light, but no. Closing my eyes again, there was now a dark blue night sky, with lots of stars.

When I finally ended the session and got up, my eyes were sore and I felt a tension, almost a pain, in the center of my forehead, in a way I have never had a soreness before.

I felt like I'd been living in this old house for 39 years, and then suddenly discovered a hidden door to a secret room. The room is big and dark, and I only have a match to light my way around. Hopefully one day, I will find the light switch, or at least a flashlight, so I can better have a look around this fascinating room.

In the fall, Debby told me we would now go on to the third phase of my healing. I had been away for three weeks on a trip to Arizona, during which my energy field had held up pretty well, despite the many trials during the trip. She explained that I now needed to get my soul back into my body, as it was not all in there.

Apparently, we leave our bodies as a way to protect the soul when the going gets too rough. It's a way to distance ourselves from too much pain. With all the events of the last few years, I am surprised my soul is even in the same room as my body! I once dated a woman who was raped repeatedly as a child. She told me she remembered parts of it from a perspective above, as if she were looking down from the ceiling. That sounds like it may have been a sort of out-of-body experience, though neither of us knew anything about that concept at the time.

To put my soul back into my body, Debby proceeded to place her hands on me and concentrate for awhile. I didn't feel anything at all. But when I tried to stand up, it felt as if the level of gravity had just doubled. I could barely walk; it was a chore just to be standing. The effect dissipated after about twenty minutes. The treatment was repeated several times, with less dramatic effect each time. I guess I was getting used to being all me in here.

Even though a lot of interesting things happened, overall progress was slow. After two months of treatment, I seemed to be worse than ever before, and then it went back to normal again. There are ups and downs while the work under the hood progresses. The apparent fast results of drugs are usually a deception that removes the symptoms, while the underlying illness continues unattended. True health takes time.

Debby prefers to do slower healings, as that is better in the long run. Some healers do fast healings, but that only removes the illness, not what caused it, so the illness may return.

One woman had been at the clinic for two months and came in a wheelchair, her husband caring for her. When they went back to Los Angeles, she was walking and her electrosensitivity had lessened to the point where she could use a computer. She credited it all to Debby.

I was spending much more than my salary could bear, and by the end of November, I had to stop all treatments and hunker down until my disability would come through. Debby was kind and gave me a free session now and then, when there was a gap in their schedule during the winter. She was clearly not in it for the money, and I was very grateful.

15

Life in the Ghetto

A routine quickly settled over my life in the Seagoville camp. I would go to Dallas twice a week, with Lawrence picking me up in the morning and driving me home late in the afternoon, before the traffic peaked.

I would see Debby each of the two days, with her team working on me. The first week I also did some allergy testing to get some more shots at Dr. Rea's clinic, but I was then advised to wait with that until more healing work had been done on me, as that could change the dosages and thus make the carefully calibrated vials a waste of money.

I did not continue the sauna treatment, as my insurance would not pay for any of it. Besides, I was living in a big sauna anyway and sweating a lot.

I did a little of intravenous infusion of vitamin B, C, Taurine, magnesium, L-Glutathione and other good stuff that made me feel really good for about two hours. It revved up my body's detoxification system, so it could get rid of whatever chemical was floating around in my blood, but it only worked as long as it kept feeding into my arm. My insurance considered it experimental and would not cover it, and I could not afford the cost. So I had to rely on the much slower and less spectacular method of taking it orally, which is much cheaper.

When I was not in Dallas, I stayed in the camp all the time. There was no other place to go at this point, without hiring someone to drive me. I could not even walk down our country road, as the residential power line along it bothered me. Besides, staying put and resting while breathing the cleaner air and maintaining my diet, allergy shots and supplements were an essential part of my program to restore my health so I could return to my home and career in Ohio.

It was like living in a ghetto, or a refugee camp, with the illness providing the walls keeping us apart from the rest of the world. We were inmates, not really free to leave. Life was very different from normal living. In a way, it was like a summer camp, where we were outdoors all day, only to go inside to sleep at night. But when did we get to go home?

112

I used to think that my most precious thing was my time. Now I had suddenly lots of it, in return for losing what was much more precious, but taken for granted — my health.

It was very hot that summer, with a record 65 days in a row with no rain at all. It was not as humid as a normal Dallas summer, and that really helped. There was an air-conditioning unit in my room, but I could not use it. Instead I spent most afternoons sitting under the big pecan tree by the pond, as that seemed to be the coolest spot in the camp.

The sun-baked un-insulated steel roof of the cook shack made it very hot in the kitchen. The refrigerators were straining against the heat, and big fans tried to move the sauna-like air around for a little comfort, with all those electrical motors spewing out lots of EMF.

My camp mates were nice to sometimes turn off the big fans in the kitchen, while I soon got my cooking down to a science of minimum exposure time inside. It only required me to be there three times: once to start it, second to turn down the heat and finally to remove the food from the burner. I ate all meals outside.

I was very glad to live in a place where I didn't constantly have to be on guard for a myriad of possible threats, such as incoming fumes from diesel trucks delivering packages, clothes dryers, barbecues, paint projects, pesticides and whatever else emanates from a typical apartment complex.

It wasn't all perfect — no place on Earth is. The large ponds surrounding the camp on three sides made the air more humid, so it was always a bit moldy, and the ponds had a musty smell to them. Dr. Rea had an allergy shot made from the water in these ponds, and that helped.

My father called me once a week to check up on me, which was a great encouragement in those dark days. I have heard many stories of how families were split by this illness, with the patient left to fend for herself when the need for help was the greatest. My family lived in Europe, so they could not be there in person, but the moral support was very tangible. I also kept in contact with friends back in Ohio, including my boss, who also provided encouragement.

I have lived in large cities all my life, so it was a change to suddenly live in a rather rural area. It was amazing how clear the sky could be at night, even with the glow from nearby Dallas. Sometimes it was possible to see the Milky Way. In the middle of August, I saw a huge shooting star move across the evening sky, with a flaming tail after it.

There wasn't much to entertain us there that summer, but it was nice to look at the nature surrounding us. A few times a big turtle would crawl across the lawn, from the front lake to the pond in the rear. It was fun to watch them fight over an apple we threw out to them in the pond. Their small mouths could not get a good grip, so the apple would just float away, with the turtle in hot pursuit.

We had several kinds of large spiders. The largest had a bright yellow body that was nearly two inches long with four-inch-long legs. The insect I found the most fascinating was the "mud dauber." It looks like a wasp, and it hunts spiders much larger than itself. It paralyzes the spider with its sting and then builds a little mud nest around it, where it places its eggs. When the eggs hatch, they have fresh meat on a silver platter. I often saw this little insect drag a much bigger spider along to where it was building its next little nest. Other times, I saw it fly along with a small spider hanging below it, like another industrial helicopter.

The first couple of months I was bothered by EMF almost everywhere in Dr. Rea's clinic. No matter where I went, it felt like the floor was vibrating. It was just a false sensation generated by my nervous system in response to the very minute radiation. It was worst in the rooms where Dr. Rea sees patients and next door where they do allergy testing. Perhaps something was going on in the offices on the floor below. I did much better in a room off the sauna area in the back of the clinic, and I often did my waiting there. The problem being in the clinic eventually simmered down, which was very encouraging.

At the Whole Foods store, the cash registers would bother me so much that I could not stand near them. Instead, I would walk right through and throw my credit card at the cashier. My respirator was a sure sign that I was environmentally ill; they were used to us so close to Dr. Rea's clinic. A few did ask in a friendly manner whether I was Dr. Rea's patient, more a statement than a question.

I avoided the Whole Foods on Preston Rd., as it was in a ritzy neighborhood with lots of fancy cars and it seemed like everybody was using their cell phones. I was several times chased around the store by cell-toting shoppers who were completely oblivious to my attempt to keep a safe distance from the radiation source.

Instead, I asked Lawrence to take me to the Whole Foods on either upper Greenville Road (it has since been closed), or one of the other stores in the area. There are some benefits to living next to a city like Dallas with many choices.

I had to use my respirator inside Whole Foods, as well as the few other stores I dared venture inside. The Whole Foods stores had a distinctive smell to them, which bothered me so much that I could smell and recognize it on the clothes of other people. I usually had to change my T-shirt after being inside a store; otherwise, the smell coming from the T-shirt was enough to make my sinuses burn.

On Friday evenings, a small company would bring groceries from Whole Foods to the camp. The owner always handled this run himself. He had spent hours inside Whole Foods before arriving and would smell so strongly that I could not be twenty feet from him. One evening he arrived so late that I was already in bed. The smell drifted in through the open window, when he passed outside, and made my head hurt. That really made me angry, but there was really nothing to do about it.

The camp had its own well, located up by the road in a little metal shack. Next to it was another shack holding a huge sand filter. It was pretty good water, though everybody drank bottled water, including the owners. Every three weeks, a truck would arrive from Mountain Valley and deliver dozens of five-gallon glass bottles. In the back of the main camp was a small concrete-block building with sturdy shelves to hold the heavy load of water. It took the poor man about an hour to haul all those bottles from his truck in the parking lot.

Like in Ohio, I had to offgas all incoming paper before I could look at it. Here it was easier as the sun was stronger and there was no rain to constantly watch for. When the mail arrived, I would don my respirator, walk to the clothesline, open each letter, hang the contents on the line and walk away. Sometimes it would still make me sick to do it, so I tried to hold my breath inside my mask. The mask is only 90 percent effective, so I still get some coming through the filters. Holding my breath didn't seem to help much. I later read in the August 2001 issue of *Our Toxic Times* that medical experiments with EI patients revealed that airborne chemicals can also reach our brain through the eyes. Other patients later showed me to use gloves when handling printed materials, to prevent them from soaking through the skin in the same way salves and skin patches work.

I didn't know any of this and was thus limited to only offgas the bare essentials of what I received. Incoming mail was rigorously sorted and any letter with an unknown return address was assumed junk mail and discarded unopened.

The most toxic type of paper I had to handle was banknotes. Banknotes contain extra chemicals for various reasons, including one that reacts with a special pen merchants can use to verify that a note is genuine. They were also frequently fragranced from people handling them.

I avoided using paper money wherever possible, but I had to pay Lawrence in cash when he drove me. Every time I got money out of the ATM, I had to hang it on the clothesline for two days. I never lost any that

I know of; people were honest and banknotes handle rain very nicely. Whoever uttered that "Money doesn't stink" definitely did not have a sensitive nose.

I got some photos developed, but they stunk terribly of the photographic chemicals. It was so strong that I couldn't spread them out on the lawn wearing my respirator but had to throw them out there, and then wait a couple of hours before I could spread them out more nicely to ensure all surfaces got aired out. And then I had to keep watch all day for the sudden gusts of wind, that would spread the pictures all over the lawn.

I got many insect bites, especially from some microscopic insect that lives in the grass and waits for a tasty "host" to walk by. Then it burrows under the skin and itches for several days. Eventually I found that covering the area with Un-petroleum Jelly (a vegetable-based alternative to Vaseline) would cut off their air supply, so the itch only lasted a day.

It is interesting that biting insects seem to prefer the sickest people. The following summer, they pretty much left me alone, while ferociously attacking the newly arrived patients. I had heard similar stories, like when someone who was environmentally ill would walk through a forest with two healthy people. Afterwards, she could count dozens of mosquito bites, while her companions would only have one or two.

Perhaps sick people send out a hormone scent or some electromagnetic signal that says, "I'm sick, take me out of the gene pool." Nature has always been good at letting predators take down the weakest specimens first. Or maybe the insects are attracted by the various chemicals that are slowly released through the pores of the skin, more so by a newly arrived person than one who has lived in a cleaner environment for some time.

The camp had a friendly dog named Daughter. She was trained to stay away from people, unless they approached her. That way people who were very allergic to dogs would not be bothered by her.

Daughter was everybody's favorite, and loved to eat leftovers. We had a rule that nobody could feed her on the patio, so she would not sit by the table and beg for food. She would be highly aggressive towards small animals—rabbits, raccoons, armadillos, skunks and small stray dogs. If a dog larger than her would enter the premises, she would be very friendly towards it. Smart dog!

She could never figure out to leave the skunks alone. Many times I would wake up at night, hearing her bark incessantly, and then the pungent odor of skunk would roll through the camp. Usually, the skunks were poor shots, but a few times they hit her, and we would have to stay clear of a very stinky dog for a few days.

She also loved to chase the rabbits. We had a lot of them, but they were too swift for her. Sometimes she would find a rabbit hole with babies in it, and then happily consume them one by one.

There were a lot of burrs in the grass, which would hang on to socks and clothes and be a menace to everybody. Daughter had learned her lesson and stayed mostly on the concrete walkways, except when chasing the smaller animals. She would then often get a burr in her paw and continue the pursuit on three legs. I once saw her get burrs on both her left paws—and continue on, using only her two right legs!

When she got a burr in her paw, she would stop and pull it out with her teeth. Once she got one on her nose, and walked around looking very pitiful. I pulled it out, and since then, she would come to me when she had a difficult burr in her paw or nose. I got a new friend!

In September, we got a new camp mate, Pam. She had gotten sick from silicone breast implants. The silicone leaked and spread throughout her body.

Every two weeks, the lawn was mowed. Nobody liked the fresh-cut grass, so we made plans in advance to be away all day, usually at Dr. Rea's clinic. Even Ellie would always run off for Dallas. The few who stayed behind would seal themselves up inside their rooms.

Around 7:40 in the morning, Jock would roll out his riding mower and briefly start the engine to warn us he meant business. Every five minutes he would start up the noisy two-cycle engine, just to make sure we didn't forget. Then at 8:00 A.M. sharp, he would drive it to the farthest corner of the lawn area and start there, while the last stragglers were hurrying out into the parking lot to get away. Manuel would follow Jock with his electric weed eater, and they would usually be finished with the many acres of turf around noon.

While I was in Ohio, I had to use my respirator so much every day that it had left a mark over the bridge of my nose. Here in the camp I could go days without using it, and the mark slowly faded away over a couple of months.

There is a distinct subculture among the environmentally ill, which is not surprising since we pretty much are restricted to our own company for socialization since the rest of the world is usually too smelly.

There are many support groups all over the country and abroad, many of which put out newsletters and also have social gatherings. Oddly enough, there was no organized group in Dallas, though there were some informal ones. Perhaps because the "population" of patients is mostly transient.

The Canadian pop-singer Kim Palmer made an album of songs about her experiences with the illness, aptly named "Songs from a Porcelain Trailer." It was very well done, with a lot of humor. I met her some years later.

We even have some expressions of our own, such as "clean," which to us means that a person or a thing or place has no odors to make people sick. The rest of the world are referred to as "normies" or "civilians," while we call ourselves "EIs" or "MCS people." Most normies are not clean and have an impaired sense of smell by the constant exposures they are subjected to, so they cannot determine whether they are clean themselves. The process of changing a lifestyle to be chemical free, and remove fragrances and other residue from clothing and belongings, is referred to as "cleaning up."

When we buy new things, we often put them outside to "offgas" the chemicals that may be embedded in them. EI homes can often be spotted by the assortment of new things that are kept outside to be seasoned, perhaps hanging on a clothesline. Before an item has been offgassed, it is "toxic," which also can refer to a person who lives the normal chemical lifestyle.

Some people are more toxic than others. Those that can be smelled easily may be referred to as a "stinker," which has nothing to do with the normal concept of proper grooming. In fact, highly groomed people are usually the worst stinkers and may even be called a "reeker." Encountering a stinker may mean we "take a hit," as we react to the plume of chemicals that surround such a person. A "reeker" is one our sensitive noses can pick up from across a street and anything they touched or sat on would stink as well.

Sometimes we may say we are "detoxing," when trying to clear chemicals from our bodies, perhaps using a sauna or supplements or simply by sweating. Chemicals, which come out of the pores of our skin and can sometimes be smelled, are referred to as being "outgassed." And when we get exposed to chemical fumes, we often become "brain fogged," an apt description that makes perfect sense to those who experience it, but is hard to explain to others. It refers to the cloudy thinking that is slowed and hard to make sense of. People who undergo chemotherapy sometimes call it "chemo-fog."

A more unfortunate concept is the "EI premium" — the fact that EIs often have to pay more, because we are sick and desperate. This is especially common in real estate, where houses that have never been pesticided or fragranced can command a premium.

Some premium is justified, as it is a specialty market. A vacant house can sit empty for a year or more, waiting for an EI who can actually afford it. There are also some special risks involved. There have been cases where

EI renters contaminated the house, making it difficult to clean up and rent out again. There have also been some investors who built or renovated houses, expecting to cash in on the premium prices, but they were not done well enough. The houses sat empty for several years, before they offgassed enough to be sold or rented out.

But there are also people who simply see desperate people as cash cows, just like some people hurry to communities devastated by natural disasters and then sell desperately needed generators and plywood at exorbitant prices.

I know multiple cases where EIs travel far to see a house, at great expense and risk to their health. When they try out the place and decide it works for them, then the price or the rent suddenly goes up by 10, 15, or 20 percent. In two cases I know, the bank refused financing a house so far above market value. In another case, it was a choice of paying or live in the car, so the guy paid.

I have seen other examples outside real estate, such as old vehicles that are sold for double their real value just because they are offgassed.

Many groups of people band together to help each other, whether they are Amish, Mormons or Freemasons. But EIs somehow seem to turn on each other when money is involved.

16

Fall 2000

The weather had been steadily hot and dry all summer. It could be completely calm all day, and then a sudden gust of wind would briefly roll through and scatter any loose piece of paper that might lie on a table. I soon learned to use rocks to hold things down, but the surprise winds still got me now and then.

The fall was still very warm, with some days topping off at 90 degrees, even into November. The nights got steadily cooler, and the day temperatures became unpredictable. Sometimes a cold front would come through and the temperature would plummet fifteen degrees in an hour or two.

In November we had several all-day rains. These were really unpleasant, as I just had to hang around under a porch roof with nothing to do. I still could not be inside the cook shack for longer periods, nor was there much else I could do besides writing letters with a pencil. I wrote a lot of letters, but I was limited by the dust from the pencil which bothered me if I stayed in my small room, and sometimes the paper would get so humid the pencil would not work on it. I lost several envelopes that glued themselves shut in the extreme humidity.

I realized that I would not be able to return to Ohio any time soon. I could not afford to continue paying the rent there and wrote a letter to six people pleading for their help in closing the apartment by October 31. They all came through wonderfully. My boss organized a work party over a weekend, where all my stuff was packed up and moved out. I was really glad I had started that job in the weeks before coming down to Texas. I had to give up the bulkier pieces of furniture as well as the stereo, which helped furnish my friend John's new house. I had just bought the used washer and dryer a few months earlier; now they went to a young family with a baby on the way, so my loss at least helped somebody out.

The smaller pieces of furniture were distributed among some of the helpers, while the crates with the smaller items were stored in my boss's barn north of the city. A few things were mailed to me, like my winter coat and my nice warm down comforter. They got the apartment cleaned up, so I got my full deposit back. That was real nice.

I was now committed to stay in Seagoville long term. There was no place for me to go back to in Ohio, and finding a new place there would be extremely difficult. The bridge back had been demolished.

Once in awhile, I would notice a whiff of a chemical odor, usually acetone, but could not figure out where it came from. It would happen without notice, and not in any particular place. It was just a quick whiff, not enough to sicken me, though it often startled me. Nobody else noticed anything, not even standing right next to me! What was going on? I finally figured out where it came from — me! After living in a cleaner environment for several months, my body had started to "clean out the attic." When my body's detoxification system was no longer able to keep up with what I got exposed to, it started to store the excess chemicals in my body fats, hoping it would later get around to breaking it down. Now my body finally got the peace from the chemical onslaught of modern living, so it could start working on the old stores. And old some of it must be, as I had not used acetone for about twenty-five years, not since I was a young teenager and loved to build plastic models. I broke my leg when I was thirteen and was holed up in my room for a couple of months. I was given a lot of airplane and ship models to glue together and paint, which I did in my little room all closed up with no ventilation during the cold northern winter. Of course, we didn't know any better, and I'll probably never know if that really had an effect on my health so many years later. It certainly didn't bother me then.

My health insurance company had a habit of "disappearing" the bills I sent to them. Dr. Rea does not take insurance — patients pay and then file with the insurance company (those of us lucky enough to have one), which then reimburses some of the money — however little they can get away with.

With my dwindling finances, it was very important to get these payments as soon as possible. A sympathetic manager at the insurance company offered that I could fax my claims directly to her desk, then she would make sure they were entered into their system. That helped greatly, but the kind woman didn't last long in that job.

I bought a small fax machine, which turned out to be a great tool for other uses as well. I quickly learned that it bothered me just like a computer, and there is in fact a microprocessor inside it. I set up the safest procedure I could to protect myself. Since I would not receive any faxes, I could remove the very stinky ribbon in it. When it was not in use, the machine resided in a plastic box on my porch.

When I needed to send a fax, I would take the machine out of the box and place it on the edge of the porch. Then I turned the power on from a distance and waited until it was ready. Then I would walk up to it, put in the paper, punch in the number and walk away. When it was done, I would turn the power off again before going near it. My exposure to the radiation was thus very brief, though I still got nailed by it if I had to hand-feed a troublesome sheet.

The biggest problem was the fact it had to be outside. It was often impossible to use it because of rain or wind. Sudden gusts of wind would often come without warning and yank the papers right out of the machine and send them flying.

I made good use of my speakerphone to keep in contact with the rest of the world. My dad called me once a week, but otherwise I did most of the calling. Sometimes I would spend hours on it during the low-fare weekends. I over-did it eventually, and started to have painful electrical symptoms, even if I stood well away from it. It was like nails were being driven into my head, accompanied by a high-pitched tone, almost as high as I could hear. My forehead would burn hours after I used the phone.

I didn't use the phone at all for a full week, to give it a rest. Then I made sure to be at least six feet away from it when I used it. That helped, but only temporarily. Slowly, I had to keep a greater distance from it to be comfortable. Fortunately, it was a very good phone I had brought with me from Ohio. It had an excellent noise-canceling microphone, so I could talk from a greater distance than with a cheaper phone.

The problem kept getting worse; I moved further away. Eventually, I reached the limit of the phone's ability to pick up my voice at twenty feet away, and it still wasn't enough. The pains in my head became excruciating, and I had to completely stop using the phone. Now I was really cut off from the rest of the world: no car, no phone, no internet, no newspapers, no television, no radio.

I kept the phone line, but would only use it very briefly. I had voicemail, which I was able to check without too much trouble, because it was a quick process. The social protocol for leaving messages does not call for the lengthy pleasantries at each end of a conversation and a lot can be said in a sixty-second message. It also allowed me to only plug the phone in once or twice a week, and get it done with. I would then reply with a letter or a postcard. The Postal Service sells cheap pre-stamped postcards with room for messages on both sides of the card. They only cost a cent above the price of the stamp. I used a lot of those. If a fast response was needed, I would send a letter by fax.

In a few cases, I got one of the other people to make the call for me.

Sometimes I would stand nearby, so messages could be relayed back and forth.

Patients usually arrive one by one at the clinic, but suddenly there were no less than three groups there. They were very different kinds of people too: seven burly truck drivers, four young nuns and some office workers. The only other groups I had heard about before were eight or ten workers who got sick while cleaning up the Exxon Valdez oil spill in Alaska, and a group of Japanese who got poisoned by the 1995 sarin gas attack in a Tokyo subway that killed 12 and injured more than five thousand.

Most of the truck drivers were big burly guys one would definitely not want to mess with. In reality they were all very nice folks with a great sense of humor that really lit up the sometimes dour climate in the clinic.

One of the biggest of these guys told me that it only took one woman, walking past him with perfume on, to make him into a quiet little mouse! Hard to believe if one has not experienced such an effect personally.

The second group was four nuns, headed by Mother Superior. They showed me pictures of their little monastery in a lush, moldy valley. The nuns had extreme mold sensitivities.

I was in the testing room with them on a slow day, when a staff member suggested that Mother Superior should try to see if she had mold allergies herself. She had just come along to chaperone the four young nuns. She reluctantly agreed, and did she get a surprise! That got her thinking, I could almost hear the wheels turn in her head while she sat next to me. She wondered out loud whether the whole monastery was getting sick from their moldy surroundings.

Over the next year, I saw a number of their nuns come through the clinic, as well as one priest. Mother Superior toured the Southwest, found a suitable property in Arizona, and moved the whole monastery, icons and all. She was quite a woman.

The third group was some office workers who had moved into a new building, with fresh paints, carpeting, etc. But the ventilation system wasn't working at all. Sick buildings cause a lot of people to get MCS.

A skunk had walked inside the cook shack one evening and stepped on a mouse trap. The poor skunk made a lot of noise trying to pry the trap off its hind leg. We didn't dare try to help it, as it would probably get afraid and spray. We just hoped it wouldn't spray the cook shack so we couldn't be in there for several days.

It finally ran out the door, with the trap still attached, much to our relief. I saw it again the following evening, limping, but without the trap.

In early November we had a big storm with a lot of water coming down, and the spectacular lightning that is so common in East Texas. The electricity went out for a couple of hours, so when the rain stopped, I went to visit a camp mate who lived in a room near the power pole. That was the first time I went inside that building since I arrived.

That storm finally broke the back on the summer, and it stayed cooler after that. The night temperatures were getting close to frost and one morning there was ice on the roads, which caused chaos in Dallas, as the Southern drivers are not used to that.

The morning lows were typically around forty degrees, while my unheated room would be about eight degrees warmer. I was very glad for my sleeping bag and thick down comforter.

Around November I started to notice that my clothes didn't seem to stink after I had been inside Whole Foods. I was always wearing a mask when I went in there, and sometimes my shirt would smell so bad I changed it when I got outside. I seemed to have gotten better, so I tried to go in without my mask. That worked. From then on, I would only use a mask when there was a problem, such as when a stinker showed up behind me in the check-out line. Of course, I paid for going unprotected many times, but I would rather do that and enjoy the anonymity.

The air quality in Whole Foods was much better than in any other store, where I still had to wear the mask, but this was a tangible improvement.

There was also an improvement with the electrical sensitivities. I noticed that the refrigerators in the cook shack were not as bad as before, and the refrigerated produce stands at Whole Foods didn't bother me at all any more. I still could not do the freezer aisle, that was still too hard.

The energy workers on Debby's team noticed the change before I said anything. They commented that some static that had always been around my head now suddenly had left and wondered if I had noticed any sudden improvement.

17

The Long Winter — Part 1

It had been a mild fall, but in November we started to have light frost on some nights, and sometimes it only warmed up to the mid-fifties in the afternoon.

The water in the ponds was still warm and generated dense fogs in the mornings, which could be very beautiful when the rays of the rising sun played through the moving clouds of mist over the water. It gave the mornings an almost mysterious feel to them, as if one could expect the Flying Dutchman to make an appearance at any time.

Migrating birds flew over in flocks on their way south. Sometimes the sky would be covered with birds for several minutes, the soft sound of thousands of beating wings filling the air. A couple of times, the flocks were so large they took a full hour to pass.

Like most EIs, I do not do as well with heat or cold as healthy people. Perhaps because my body temperature is unstable, and always low. On any given day, it could vary between 95 and 98 degrees. Rarely would it reach the normal 98.6 degrees.

I was not able to run the electric heater while inside my room, so it was often in the low forties on those cold mornings, and I slept fully clothed.

On one of the first days in December, we had very pleasant weather, reaching seventy degrees in the afternoon. Two of us put up strings of Christmas lights on the corrugated steel wall of the cook shack. We wanted the place to look at least a little like the Christmas season.

The weather forecast warned of dramatically colder weather the next afternoon. In the evening it was still balmy, and the next morning it was a surprisingly warm 63 degrees. Then the temperature started dropping, as I noticed the wind turning from the south to the north. Within the hour, the temperature had dropped ten degrees and by eleven it was down to 43 degrees.

Sue took off for Dr. Rea's clinic around noon, driving my car with me in the back seat. I needed to deliver a lab test, do some paperwork and then just intended to hang out in the warmth for the rest of the day.

While I sat in the main waiting room, I noticed three Germans, who were talking to a clinic staff member about their housing problems. They had arrived from Germany the night before and not done well in the clinic housing. The staffer knew me and asked if I would tell them about where I lived, as perhaps that would work better for them.

The patient was a young woman named Renate (not her real name), who had flown over with her mother and a friend.

After I told them about the place I lived, they decided to stay there for the night. They had arranged for a rental car, and a woman from the rental agency arrived just then to pick them up. While the Germans got ready to go, the rental agent asked me what kind of place this clinic was. When I briefly explained, she told me that she had headaches all the time, except when she rented a cabin in the country. I heard that sort of thing a lot.

Renate stayed at the clinic, while the two others went to the car agency to do the paperwork and pick up the car. I had already done what I came for, so I spent the time with Renate. She had many questions and seemed disappointed in the clinic setup, especially that some people wore fragrances. Her face and arms were covered with red marks from her reactions, and she was obviously not feeling well. Her mouth and nose were covered by a ceramic mask, which was connected to the oxygen tank with a flexible steel pipe. Despite it all, there was sparkle and intelligence evident in her clear blue eyes.

When a woman walked by, her fragrances rolling over us, I put on my own mask and then watched how Renate's clear eyes became bloodshot within a minute. It was as if someone had punched her — the whites turned all red.

I understood her puzzlement that this could happen here. In the German culture, the signs asking people to come without fragrances would be heeded, but, for better or worse, nobody can tell an American what to do.

Her two companions returned after an hour, and we all took off. Renate rode with Sue and I, as my car was much safer than their rental car. The others followed in their car.

We first went to the small health food store called Roy's Market. Sue needed to buy a few things and Renate was famished. She was so limited in what she could eat and had had very little since they left Germany.

The temperature had kept dropping throughout the day, and it was now below freezing with a chilly wind, making it very unpleasant to be outside. Renate preferred to stay outside anyway, rather than go inside the store or wait in the car. I kept her company, while the rest did their shopping. Besides all her other problems, she also had problems tolerating clothing and she didn't have a coat to protect her from the cold wind, only a padded blanket, which was draped over her thin frame.

While we were waiting outside, we were passed by a woman who hurried to her car, only wearing shorts and a blouse. I commented on her bravery and she laughed that the change of weather had caught her by surprise — it had been seventy the day before, after all.

It was a cold wait, but finally they all came back out and we drove out to the camp. It took us forty-five minutes to get there in the rush-hour traffic, and we arrived at six, as it was getting dark.

Ellie had been notified of the new arrivals and had made two rooms ready and warm. She hadn't been told that Renate was electrically sensitive, and the rooms were near the incoming power-line, so Renate had to be moved to another room, which was bitterly cold.

I went to cook dinner for myself in the cook shack, and soon Renate's mother came to cook for the three of them. All the shared cookware was of steel, which Renate couldn't handle, so I lent them one of my glass pots and someone else lent them a wooden spoon.

The weather was forecasted to go down to around twenty degrees, so Ellie decreed that we had to have the electrical heaters on all night, and let the water faucets run, to prevent the pipes from freezing. This was a big problem for me, as there was no way I could be inside my little room with an electrical heater running.

First I decided to sleep on the concrete floor in the cook shack, as far away from the heaters and refrigerators in there as possible. It would be a big exposure and I was concerned about getting more sensitive — it was difficult enough as it was. And it was possible to get worse.

Another possibility was to sleep in the concrete block building where we store the water bottles, but it too had to be heated that night.

At eleven at night, I finally decided to try sleeping in my tent. I have camped many times in cold weather, but not this cold. I put up my three-season tent so my little hut would break the wind. My sleeping bag was rated for twenty degrees, but those ratings are always quite optimistic and during the twelve years of use, it had lost a lot of the insulation value. I climbed in fully clothed, wearing a sweatshirt and my winter coat. I put my down comforter on top of the sleeping bag. That ought to do it.

I woke up feeling cold around four in the morning. I was not in danger of hypothermia, but I stayed awake and stirred to stay warm enough. By eight, I climbed out and got some breakfast. We had 19 degrees that night, besides the wind chill. Not a picnic.

It only warmed up to 34 degrees during the day, while the bitterly cold wind continued to come down from the north. The next night did not look promising.

I called Dolores, who had a house in Seagoville where she rents out rooms to people with MCS. She did not like renters who are electrically sensitive, as she then couldn't watch TV or do other things she liked, but she agreed to let me stay for a night or two. She had lived six years in the camp, so she knew what it was like.

I quickly ate my dinner and drove over there. The windshield was covered with ice, but it was easy to remove. The road was still warm and the ice didn't stay on it. I had to have the headlights on, which doubled the electrical emissions in my car, so I was glad when the seven-minute ride was over.

Dolores's house had four bedrooms around a formal living room. The floors were all covered with ceramic tiles, and in some rooms the walls were covered with aluminum foil to seal in fragrances that were embedded in the porous drywall — a leftover from the previous owner's use of "plug-in" fragrance dispensers.

A central air handling system cleans the air with charcoal filters and cools the air during the summer, while electric space heaters are used throughout the house during the winter.

The attached two-car garage had been converted to a large kitchen and lounge for the renters. The garage doors were replaced with large sliding-glass doors, making it the cheeriest place in the whole house, which otherwise only had few and small windows.

This extra kitchen allowed Dolores to have her own private kitchen, and keep cooking odors out of the house. It is also the social center, where her renters would usually spend their day.

I was the only guest that night, though she expected a woman from Pennsylvania shortly, and another a few weeks later.

One of the bedrooms had been painted six months earlier and was still being aired out. The window to the room was kept open all the time and the door to the room was sealed with aluminum tape to keep the fumes out of the house.

I was issued a small bedroom with a bed, but no mattress. It was a bit stuffy in there, so I let it air out a little and left the space heater off for the night. I camped on the floor, luxuriating in indoor comfort.

By noon it had warmed up outside, and water was streaming off the roof. My car was still covered in ice, but it was melting and the road was already dry. The weather forecast promised nightly lows around thirty, so I drove home again.

The three Germans had moved back to Dallas and found another of the clinic condos that was better. They had considered giving up and flying back to Germany right away, but now they were able to stay for some weeks, as planned.

My neighbor in the other side of the little duplex moved to a house shortly before Christmas. I was happy for him. It also made my life easier, since his activities often prevented me from being inside my room during the day. He was a nice guy and had his needs, so there wasn't anything to do about it.

In the evening a group of Christmas carolers came from a church and sang for us. The dozen singers sang for half an hour and then a prayer was conducted, before they continued on their tour visiting people who were sick and homebound. That was very nice.

Ellie and Jock went around on Christmas Eve and gave each of us a small glass sculpture. Mine was a beautiful glass apple, which I have been using as a paperweight ever since.

Christmas Day was cold and rainy, one of those really-hard-to-get-out-of-bed days, where the temperature in my room was only in the thirties. A couple of us were invited to attend a Christmas dinner in Dallas, so we got to escape the dreary camp for the afternoon.

The party was held at one of the clinic condos, one that was well away from the big power-line at the end of the complex and I did fine for the four or five hours we were there. It was a great party, attended by a dozen long-term patients, who had kept in contact since we all arrived in the fall of 1999, a year ago. It was a diverse group, including a physician, a retired Hollywood actress, the owner of a construction company and the woman who cleans these condos.

The food was wonderful: turkey with all the trimmings and great desserts. It was even the proper day on my rotation diet for most of it, though I would have cheated otherwise.

Two of the other patients had strong food reactions and one of them so much she nearly collapsed and had to use an oxygen mask.

For a precious few hours, we were warm and comfortable, ate good food and were surrounded by cheerful people. We could forget the realities of our daily lives. Many of us had improved our health over the past year, some very visibly so.

The next day was also cold and drizzly, still not making it to forty degrees outside. I stayed in my bed all day, no reason to go outside other than to eat. Inside was only a few degrees warmer than outside, but there was no wind.

The highlights of these cold days were the meals and the daily bath. I filled the tub with water as hot as I could tolerate, and stayed in it until it got cool. It lost its heat too fast, being in a room that was only a few degrees above freezing. The steam coming off the water created a dense fog in the tiny bathroom and made the cold steel walls glisten with condensation.

The kitchen provided little relief. Its walls and ceiling were just sheets of corrugated steel plates without any insulation. With four big space heaters going, 6000 watts of heat, it didn't even get to sixty degrees in there. The electrical bill must be horrendous. I estimate that there were about 25 kilowatts of space heaters going on such a day.

Early in the winter, Jock and Ellie would only allow two space heaters in the kitchen, to save electricity. Someone figured a crafty solution to that by developing a constant craving for baked potatoes— potatoes that needed to be baked for many hours. Jock or Ellie would sometimes come to check that we were not using more space heaters, but they never wizened up to this little subterfuge.

Sue and Pam were now the only other people using the kitchen. They spent much of their day inside the cook shack and were nice to turn off the heaters so I could be inside to cook and eat. The first month we used the heaters, I was fine with two of them running in the far end of the kitchen, but that didn't last.

Without the heaters on, it didn't take long before the kitchen got chilly and they wanted the heaters back on again, so it was time to go. While I was in the cook shack, I had turned on a space heater in my room so it felt pleasant when I returned, but that luxury only lasted about an hour.

The clinic was open again on the 27th. Sue and I drove in there to be benchwarmers and socialize with the other patients. There were a lot of people sitting around that day, as a gas pipeline had ruptured in the street outside the condo complex. The rupture may have been caused by the construction work for the new DART light-rail commuter line they were constructing.

The billboards along the freeway showed 29 degrees when we drove home in the dark, and another deep freeze was forecast for the night. We had to have the heaters on again in our rooms, but this time I could sleep in the recreation room that was now vacated.

The recreation room had a raw concrete floor, directly on the ground, so it was warmer than my own room, which had a steel floor with wooden floorboards and about two feet of open airspace beneath it.

I used this room for these frosty nights for the remainder of my stay in the camp and even considered moving into it, but realized it would be problematic in the hot summers as there were two close neighbors who both used air-conditioning.

It snowed on the last day of the year and it was all white for a couple of days. On the fourth day of the new year it warmed up again and we could bask in a few afternoons in the sixties, before it went down to the thirties and forties for the rest of the month.

The meteorologists declared this to be the coldest December in seven years—nothing compared to a winter in Ohio, but it felt colder with these living arrangements. A camp like this would probably not be feasible in a northern climate. This was Sue's second New Years here, and she told us that the previous year it had been so warm that they had walked around in T-shirts and set up a TV outside to watch the millennium celebrations.

I developed a system to minimize the time I needed to be inside the cook shack, to save precious heat for when I was ready to sit down and eat. Pam and Sue also often used the ovens, which were a bit much for me too. I would first turn the burner for my pot up on high, then leave and come back four minutes later. I would then turn it down and leave until the food was done, twenty minutes later. I carried a mechanical wind-up clock in my pocket to keep me right on time.

The others used the cook shack as their living room, and sometimes read magazines in there, which emit fumes that were a problem for me. They were nice to keep them closed while I was in there. In return, I did similar things for them or carried heavy things for them.

In early November, I figured out a way for me to read books. Sue received meat shipments from the Welsh Family Farms in Iowa in heavy clear plastic bags. I hung one of them up to offgas for several days and then put an open book inside, together with an unsharpened pencil. The bag was then sealed air tight. I could then safely read the open book through the plastic bag. To turn the page, I grabbed the pencil through the plastic and used the eraser head to gently flip the page.

This was a godsend, especially when confined to my bed on cold days. I had not been able to read anything for a year, so I really went for it. While I was working, I rarely had time to read anything that was not related to my profession, so now I made up for that by only reading more frivolous stuff, such as the Shogun novels and stories by Tom Clancy. That joy only lasted three months, then disaster struck and I got sensitized to the plastic. I had been careful to air them out first, but plastic never really airs out—if the plasticizers are all offgassed, the plastic becomes hard and brittle. Now I had gotten so sensitive that I got dizzy, even if sitting outside with it. I could even smell the plastic bags now, a pretty good indicator of sensitization.

Other types of plastic became problematic at the same time. I didn't have much, but some old sheet protectors and three-ring binders had to go. The worst problem was that I no longer could tolerate my old sleeping bag but would wake up with a thundering headache every morning. It was twelve years old, but that was no longer enough for me to tolerate the nylon and synthetic fill.

I had been sleeping in my sleeping bag, with a thick down comforter and a blanket on top. To compensate for the loss of the sleeping bag, I would instead bring two or three gallon-size glass bottles with hot water to bed with me. That was very nice, better than the sleeping bag.

The problem with the sleeping bag could have been dust mites. They had given me problems before, but washing and hanging it up for some frost treatment did not improve things.

Now I had nothing to do on the days I stayed in bed. I was tired of counting all the screws that held together the steel plates covering the ceiling, walls and floor. Then I thought of going for long walks in my memory and spent hours wandering the halls of my childhood school buildings, cities I have visited and the like. My long-term memory seemed to work pretty well.

I passed a lot of time writing many letters to my parents, letters that later formed the basis for this book. My dad wrote me back at least once a week. He wrote mostly about their daily life, people they met, places they went, just normal life that still existed but seemed so far away. Sometimes I imagined that I could just walk out of there and everything would be normal again, nothing bad would happen if I did what everybody else could do. Maybe one day...

In the spring I came up with an improvement to my reading bag system. Instead of a plastic bag, I used a cellophane bag. It was a laborious system; the cellophane bags were not roomy and they sprung leaks. To turn the page, I grabbed the pencil gently through the cellophane, wedging it in under the next page. Sometimes I had to roll it in under, using the eraser head to get enough traction to move the sheet a little, then push the pencil in under it. Then, lift up a bit — check the page number. If I got hold of two pages, I had to start over. Once I got the right page, I would slowly push the page with the pencil, sometimes jiggling the bag or shoving the book around inside. Ah, there. Oops, the smell of ink and mold might then suddenly appear. Then I had to find the leak, the little rip that had formed, and patch it up with a small piece of aluminum tape.

Eventually, the bag would get so worn that it would leak every time I turned a page. By then, there were dozens of patches in it, especially around the edges and the lower-right corner where I grabbed the pencil. And I could no longer find all the tiny, tiny leaks that together started to add up. It often took two bags to read one book, and they cost a dollar apiece. I still got nailed by the leaking fumes on and off, but it was allowing me to read some.

18

Disability Circus — Act 1

When I had been two months in Texas, I realized it was a good idea to look into what disability coverage I had and get the information together. In retrospect, I should have started much earlier, as it took months before the application could even be sent off. A whole month was wasted just getting the proper forms. But it was not a thing I was ready to consider sooner; it was a big change to think of not working at all.

My employer assigned a case manager to help me. She was a great help and encouragement. I sent her some information about the illness, including a copy of the picture book *The Dispossessed* by Rhonda Zwillinger, which very graphically describes the lifestyle imposed upon us, through fifty pictures. I was concerned that she would not believe me, but she did and told me that she had actually worked on a case stranger yet.

I was not eligible for Social Security, but I was covered by two overlapping disability policies. The primary policy, which I shall refer to as SERP, pays more and includes a health plan. The secondary, FERIT, pays less and has no health plan. If both plans accepted me, SERP would basically take over. She recommended I apply to both. The applications were nearly identical anyway.

We started building the case, and there were many forms to fill out. I had to get statements from my management, from Social Security, my doctors and myself. I also needed a copy of my birth certificate.

Dr. Rea also recommended a neuropsychological evaluation, which took place in early September. There were a lot of papers to be filled out, and the ink fumes were a problem, so I was not at my best. Of course, I never really felt good, so it wasn't that much of a difference.

It was a long, tiring day, with many questions and many types of tests. My psychological state of mind was probed; my sense of balance was tested. My short- and long-term memory skills were checked, as were my mathematical, logical and general problem solving skills. Even my coordination was inspected.

The memory tests were hard for me, much harder than I had expected. The long-term memory worked splendidly, but short-term memory was a problem. That really made it hit home how my brain had been affected, more than the dizziness that came and went, depending on how safe the air I breathed was.

I was told sequences of numbers, that I then had to repeat back. I failed miserably there, but then she gave me simple math problems, which I could do at a rate well above the average, as one should expect from a computer engineer. At least that worked well.

The final report was very detailed and very thorough, pointing out how I compared with average men of my age group and education in various ways. It was well worth the expense.

The two disability plans later hired several physicians to look at the documentation, and when I later got to see their reports, it was clear that this neuropsychological test was the one nobody dismissed.

I got a nice four-page letter from Dr. Rea in support of my case, and his legendary patient educator, Carolyn Gorman, suggested getting a letter from a second doctor as well. She recommended Dr. A., so I went to see him.

Lawrence dropped me off early for my appointment with Dr. A. I had the first appointment of the day and had some time to do grounding work first. Riding with Lawrence usually loaded me up with a charge, even though I always sat in the back seat, where the radiation was minimal.

I walked over to a small tree to the side of the building and used it for my grounding. That allowed me to do it very inconspicuously, instead of lying down on the ground. When I was done, I went inside.

Dr. A. was a very likable person. He asked me to tell my story, and he really meant it. For a full hour, he basically listened and took notes. I had wondered whether I should tell him the full truth, including about my electrical sensitivities, but I felt comfortable with this man and did. At the end, he quietly told me that he had arrived early that morning himself and sat outside on a bench, noticing the grounding work I did with the tree! Only a person who understood what I was doing would have noticed anything unusual going on. He wrote me a very nice letter.

The whole package with my disability application was finally ready and shipped out late in October. My case manager in Ohio had looked it over first and found the level of documentation impressive. She was enthusiastic about my prospects and thought it might go through in about three months. That turned out to be very optimistic.

My accumulated vacation and sick leave finally ran out in December, having carried me since I crashed in May. Now I had no income, and my savings had already taken a beating with all the medical expenses over the last couple of years. My parents started to send me money, but they were not able to even cover the rent. At least I still had medical coverage, as the place I worked for had a very generous policy of providing coverage for a full year, for people in the process of applying for disability. That was a very humane thing to do and really ought to become the norm, but sadly it isn't.

I had already stopped all treatments and now trimmed my expenses to the bare necessities, while waiting for my case to be pondered. If they took their time, I would have to start eating my pension.

In January, I was notified by my primary plan that they would send me to be seen by a physician in Dallas, who would evaluate my case. They used an agency which provided doctors for such evaluations, court cases, etc. I was relieved they would not try to force me to go back to Ohio.

I still couldn't use the phone, so Sue called the doctor's office and got them to mail me their questionnaire. That way I could offgas it and answer the questions ahead of time, so it would not affect me even before I met the doctor.

I wrote a short and friendly letter directed to the receptionist, asking if it was possible that the doctor could refrain from using any cologne or other fragrances on the day of my visit, and perhaps also avoid wearing freshly laundered clothes. The day before the appointment, I called her myself, asking if she had received the letter, and if there were any questions. I was simply told that I could discuss it with the doctor when I got there. I was still so naive in the ways of doctors.

I was determined to keep my head clear as much as possible, so I wore my respirator throughout the visit. I did sample the air in the waiting room, which smelled a little of carpet chemicals, though wasn't terrible. Worse was that the place was loaded with electromagnetic radiation, though I could not see where it came from. I figured there must be a lot of computers and other equipment behind the flimsy walls or on the floor below. I walked around the waiting room, feigning interest in what was on the walls, to try to find a comfortable area. There was none — I just had to endure it. The area around the elevator seemed a little better, so I developed a great interest in the view out of the window there.

After I had been there twenty minutes, an upbeat assistant led me into a tiny examination room. I noticed there was a PC right outside the door, with nobody using it. She happily turned it off. Inside the room, a speaker in the ceiling blasted elevator music rather loudly; she cheerfully turned it down. I was still very uncomfortable with EMF symptoms and saw nothing else to do about it, besides disconnecting a battery charger for the instrument the doctor used to look inside the ears and the nose. I did that while the assistant was away and I was alone.

Then Dr. B. arrived. He was courteous but not friendly. There was no warmth to him except when I praised his staff at the end. Then he did crack a nice smile.

He allowed me to speak freely for no more than a minute, then he only allowed me short responses to his questions. I was feeling steadily worse in there, with a loud ringing in my ears, pains in my chest area and a burning sensation in my legs— symptoms from high EMF exposures. My mind was also unclear, so I was basically just able to keep responding to his questions. I had brought a sheet with me with talking points, because I expected problems, but I even forgot I had it on my lap.

I continued to feel worse in there. At the end, my legs felt like they were smoldering with fire. I am sure hot-dogs could have been roasted on my bare skin, but I was determined not to say anything, as he then surely would consider me crazy. I had made that strong decision ahead of time, and stuck to it. My blood pressure is typically 100/75, with the highest ever measured at Dr. Rea's being 128/62 on a really lousy day. Dr. B's assistant measured it at 130/80 at the start of the session; wonder what it was at the end. As dimwitted as I felt, it amazes me that I could recall so much the next day to write detailed notes, but that is an effect I have noticed several times.

Dr. B. then looked in my mouth and up my nose. The interview was clearly winding down and I had a strong feeling that a lot was unsaid, though my sheet with the talking points was still forgotten. I then remembered that I had to give him copies of the lab reports and a form to fill out, as instructed in the stern letter from the agency. It turned out that they had sent him a set themselves, so my insistence on giving it to him probably annoyed him as it took me awhile to realize it. At this point, I was definitely not mentally fit to drive a car.

Amazingly, I did remember to plug the battery charger back in before I left. Dr. B. did notice it was disconnected during the interview, as he mentioned it in his report.

I had been inside the building for ninety minutes and was exhausted when I got down on the street again. I simply laid myself on the concrete walkway to rest and try to get rid of the electrical charge I could feel pulsing through my body. Perhaps like when people are hit by a phaser beam on *Star Trek*, and are engulfed in a luminous glow for awhile after. I would not have been too surprised to actually see sparks flying off me.

I was definitely not able to get rid of this fire on my own. I had not been in so much pain since I arrived in Dallas. I staggered over to Dr. Rea's clinic and was lucky to see one of Debby's apprentices. She worked on me right away and got it simmered down. By that evening, I felt like I had recovered fully from the onslaught.

I was surprised that Dr. B's office was that bad. I will never know for sure what the problem was, but some months later I happened to see the building from a distance, and noticed that there were several cell phone transmitter pods located on the roof of the building, perhaps thirty or forty feet from where I had been.

When I finally got to see a copy of the report three months later, it was an interesting read. He concluded that my symptoms do seem to correlate with the diagnosis of MCS but that MCS is highly controversial and not supported by any evidence that he was willing to accept. He could not support my case and suggested that I might be disabled on psychological grounds, since I clearly believed my own story.

The next I heard was a written summons to be interviewed by a psychiatrist, a Dr. C. Two days later, I received a friendly handwritten note, with a questionnaire to be filled out. It asked many questions about suicide tendencies, how much I drink, use illegal drugs, etc, etc. Many pages of questions that didn't pertain to me. The note also stated that I would need to plan on spending three hours in his office!

With the ninety-minute torture at Dr. B's office fresh in mind, I decided to request an accommodation to be seen elsewhere. Dr. Rea was doubtful that such a request would be honored but agreed to write the request, with the offer that we could meet at Dr. Rea's clinic. It was not far from Dr. C's office, so it didn't seem like an outlandish request. The letter also suggested that he arrive unscented.

The time was very short. I was only given two weeks' notice for the meeting, which was to be held the first week of April. I decided to write a note to Dr. C., advising of the letter that would follow. Then I tried to call the agency, as the summons letter sternly stated that no changes in the appointment could be made without the approval of a named person. When I asked for the person listed in the letter, it was clear that I had asked for God himself. And He did not talk to lowly beings like me. I was then switched to another person, who did not make me feel any more welcome. She told me that if I had already met one of their doctors in his office, I could do it again, though if my doctor could make a case, they would consider it. It was very clear that such a request was quite unlikely to be looked upon favorably.

Dr. Rea's overburdened secretary produced the letter in a week and it was quickly faxed and mailed to both Dr. C. and the agency. I hadn't received any response the day before the interview, so I called Dr. C's office. He answered himself and was very dismissive. In an overbearing tone, he informed me that he had lost all interest in the case. Apparently, I was too much trouble for his Lordship. He had canceled the appointment, but nobody had bothered to inform me. SERP followed up with a letter that was a flat denial of my request, and it basically stated that I would show up at the next appointment I would be summoned for and see the doctor inside his office.

The next summons arrived speedily. This piece of absurd theatre only produced a three-week delay in the process.

Dr. D's office cheerfully mailed me their questionnaire when asked, but otherwise I didn't dare ask or say anything. I'd rather not know in advance if they intended me to stay there for a lengthy period as well.

The questionnaire had a lot of the same questions, such as whether I abused coffee, alcohol, tobacco, etc., and the usual ones about how many (other) crazy people there were in my family. Then there were a lot of questions about symptoms, such as whether I had headaches, difficulty concentrating, tingling sensations or if I ever avoided specific locations or situations. No wonder some of these people think we are nuts—we fit nicely into some of their little templates.

Dr. D's office was spartan, and the air quality fairly good, though I kept my mask on to keep my mind clear.

Dr. D was pleasant and attentive, allowing me to speak freely and asked intelligent questions. He seemed to have an understanding of what I talked about and even knew that detergents and fragrances could make people sick.

Late in the session, he quickly went through a series of standard questions, like who was the current president, the capital of Texas and such. I was also given a few memory tests, which I did fair on, I think. I felt fine in there, my head was clear, and with Dr. D's positive attitude it was a good experience.

I expected the report to say that I was not a psychiatric patient and that my problems were outside his field of expertise, perhaps suggesting that I be evaluated by a more appropriate specialist. So I waited for another summons. Two months later, I got disappointed when I received a flat denial of my case.

Dr. D's report had indeed cleared me of psychiatric disease, but then only went on to state that although I am supported by two doctors and a

Ph.D.-psychologist, the report from Dr. B stated that there is no objective evidence for my case. The agency clearly took their "own" doctor's evaluation as gospel. The denial letter simply stated that "there was not significant objective evidence of a disabling condition." It then proceeded to inform me of the appeal process, including the strict deadlines. I ended up using all the available time, including the filing extension, with only a few days to spare.

The rejection was not a terrible surprise, as I had already heard from many that a rejection of the first filing is pretty much standard in the industry. A sort of cruel extra screening to weed out those who are not truly desperate. At the time of this writing, I have only heard of very few people who were approved by Social Security, or any other system, in the first round. One of these people had a U.S. senator to actively support her case. Most of the success cases were in the last couple of years. Perhaps we are gaining some acceptance.

People who have already exhausted their financial means may not be able to mount an appeal at all. Documentation costs money, lots of money. And if the appeal is also denied, which most are, then it costs a lot of money to hire a lawyer. Even lawyers working on a contingency basis often want some money upfront as well.

Some people simply give up and become a burden to their families, perhaps becoming homeless, never having a chance to live a life under humane conditions. It is not a system with fairness in it, as the cards are clearly stacked, though most people eventually do win.

I had no choice but to mount an appeal. There was no other option. The problem was that I was living off my fast dwindling savings, with some help from my family. My rent cost was high, with no cheaper place available I would be able to live in. I couldn't even move into my car, as I was unable to drive it. It was not even street legal any more, as the Ohio plates had expired and it would cost a lot to do the necessary repairs and registration fees.

I tried to wrack my brain to find some way to make money, but when I couldn't handle a car, a phone, a computer, papers and many other substances, besides rarely being clear headed, I was very limited. The best idea I came up with was to be a night watchman for one of the gravel quarries in the area. That would require me to sleep in the day, which was impossible in the noisy camp.

I was getting ready to start eating my pension fund, when the white knight arrived.

For months, I had pretty much ignored the secondary disability plan.

They had not asked for any more information or sent me to be examined by any doctor.

They did send all the lab work to a doctor, a specialist in occupational health, who wrote a very long and detailed report. He straddled the fence, on one side saying that there was objective evidence of impairments and abnormalities, while also saying that the diagnosis was controversial and not well supported. They did approve me! The notice arrived less than a month after the primary plan denied my claim.

19

The Long Winter — Part 2

Jock died suddenly in January.

Of immediate concern was whether Ellie would be able to continue running the camp on her own or if she would need to close it down, making us homeless. Finding another place to live would be extremely difficult; there simply was no backup plan. Before Jock's body was even removed, Ellie came over to the rest of us and assured us that she would keep the place open. Nobody had asked her. Despite her grief, she was able to think of our concerns.

Right behind my room was a little metal shed with a washer and dryer. It was used exclusively to wash bedding when people moved out. We were issued seven cotton pads to sleep on, two towels and two blankets. It is up to the resident to wash them as needed, but we were not required to return them freshly laundered. It had been one of Jock's jobs to wash these, but he had fallen far behind. The little shed was piled up high with unwashed bedding. I had been glad he ran behind, because the machines bothered me when they ran, so I could not be in my room.

When Ellie started working on the piles, she often started the machines at an inconvenient time for me. A few times, she started them late in the evening, so I had to abandon my warm bed and go out in the rain to wait it out. I suggested that I do the laundry. She was not enthusiastic but let me do it, and on my schedule.

Starting the washer was easy, as it just starts by filling the tumbler. But the dryer would start running the electric motor and the heating elements right away, which bothered me. I solved the problem by using a large broomstick to push the start button. To stop the machines, I could just flip the breaker on a pole outside the shed. I used the clotheslines whenever possible, to minimize the use of the dryer and not waste energy.

Now I no longer had to anxiously lie in my bed, listening to Ellie's footsteps on the concrete walkway. Waiting to hear whether she would just pass by on another errand, or walk into the little shed and perhaps start one of the machines. And it helped her out, making it more feasible to keep the place open.

Late in January, we got a new camp mate. Joanne (not her real name) was a very sad and afraid person when she was brought over. She had a hard time adjusting to camp living. She had trouble tolerating the trailer she moved into and she had to work on getting her clothes free of fabric softener and other stuff they'd picked up. Her cooking habits were a problem for the rest of us, as she fried her foods and used strong spices, which made it difficult to share the kitchen with her. Pam finally chewed her out over it, which Joanne took very hard. When she started burning vegetables on the stove, to make digestive charcoal, the smoke even bothered me on my porch and I had to complain too. Joanne then borrowed a portable hotplate and did these things on her own porch.

What was more disturbing was that she confided in me that she was tired of this ragged life. She wanted to commit suicide, preferably with my help! I was able to talk her out of it, with some help from Dr. Cole, a psychotherapist who is associated with Dr. Rea's clinic. It was difficult communicating with Dr. Cole, as I could not use the phone, so a number of notes were mailed, faxed and hand carried by Sue. I was glad when that calmed down again. When I got to know Joanne better, I could see that she was not really serious, but desperate — the ultimate cry of despair. Later she even joked about it, like when during the next summer we had a patient who was rushed to the emergency room in an ambulance. Joanne's comment was that she had planned to commit suicide that day, but this commotion stole all the attention, so she had decided to wait for a better day. This sort of humor may be difficult to understand for outsiders.

Almost all EIs contemplate suicide at some point or other. I knew the situation of the suicides that had already happened, and the ones to follow, and in their situation I would probably have done the same. Fortunately, I have never been close enough to actually plan it, but simply knowing that I could go through with it, and not give any hint to other people, gave me a sense of peace to get through those winter months and the first year in Dallas. I knew it would not have to be like this forever — there was always at least one way out.

To me, it seems perverted that one does not have the right to end one's own life, and the state will spend enormous effort to prevent it, but so little is really done to help people come away from their hopeless situation, whether it is serious illness, mental illness, disability, deep poverty or other depraved situations.

Depression is common among EIs as it is for many groups of patients whose lives have been drastically altered and have chronic symptoms. On top of that, the brain chemistry of EI patients is often altered by the toxic chemicals that have been stored in the brain — the body's largest deposit of fatty tissues. This can then result in other common problems, such as sleeplessness and anxiety.

Fortunately, I don't seem to have those problems myself, and I sleep well at night. Fellow patients have often commented that I seem unusually cheerful for an EI. I just try to make the best of the present situation and hope for better times, instead of giving up. I also had a growing sense that there is more to life than it seems, as brought home to me that day when Debby with her incredible abilities pulled me out of a very painful situation that could have ended in my death. I'm too curious not to stick around, if for no other reason.

A friend of Joanne's drove her car down and flew back home. It held the last few possessions she had, including a toaster oven, a water distiller, a tiny black-and-white television, a couple of books and a pogo stick. Some day, someone should write a thesis about what things people end up with, when they have to get rid of most of their possessions. It could be quite interesting.

Joanne had started sauna treatment at the clinic, and soon her body started to outgas various chemicals through her pores. We all do this to some degree. On a warm day, I could sometimes still smell a whiff of acetone coming out of me. But Joanne was emitting a lot, and constantly. I was particularly bothered by whatever came out of her and had to keep a good distance. It permeated all her clothes and belongings, so when she washed her clothes, I had to stay clear of the cookshack where the washers were and keep at least forty feet away from the trailer she lived in — even if she was not there. Her car also smelled of this chemical cocktail. The smell was unpleasant to the other camp mates, but it didn't make them sick as it did me.

This stage lasted about a month. Then she cut down on her sauna treatments, as they were hurting her — going too fast. She nearly collapsed one day in the sauna and was sick for several days after. When she cut down her sauna treatments, the outgassing would only happen in spurts, and over the next couple of months it died down. By then the fumes would be more varied and no longer made me sick. Sometimes she smelled like a pharmacy, remnants of all the drugs a legion of doctors had filled her with over the years. With her body unable to break down the synthetic drugs, it had just stored them in her fatty tissues to be dealt with later.

The only other male resident of the camp during the winter was a guy whom we never saw. He rarely ventured outside his little camper and never talked to anyone. I shared the cook shack with the three women for the latter part of the winter, and sometimes had to hear them complain about their loneliness and lack of romantic companionship. I got hold of a card with a picture of a skeleton woman sitting on a park bench with her skeleton poodle, under the headline: "waiting for Mr. Right." I hung it up in the kitchen on Valentines Day, and it was promptly removed. It hit a little too close to home.

A camp mate cut her finger with the kitchen knife one evening, and put a band-aid on it. The plastic smell of the band-aid bothered her, so the next couple of days she wore a cotton glove on the hand to close in the fumes. Life in our world sure is different.

I walked around the camp a lot, in great circles, on the concrete walkways. This was both to stay warm, for exercise and plain boredom. I would often go up on a small protrusion into the front pond, which we called "the bluff," even though it was only a foot higher than the area behind it. I could sometimes hear some strange chewing-like sounds at night, but would not be able to see anything. A few times I seemed to see something swim in the dark water, but that was all. Finally, in the last light of the day, I saw a beaver swim around. When it spotted me, it immediately gave a warning flap with its tail and dived out of sight. That made my day.

January was a cold dark month to get through. Since I only had a flashlight in my room, I pretty much had to go to bed when it got dark outside, as there wasn't anything else to do. I could only be inside the kitchen for brief visits, before it got too cold and the heaters had to be put back on. Some days were cold and rainy, so I had to spend most of the time in my bed to stay comfortable. I was glad when February arrived. The days were longer, though the weather wasn't much better, except during the first week. We then had several balmy days with blue skies and about seventy degrees, until King Winter decided to show he wasn't beaten yet. I was awakened by a storm at 1 A.M. and went outside to check the things on my porch. I stored most of my things in large plastic buckets and a steel trash can, which were waterproof. But I also had a number of magazines and other things laying in the open to be offgassed. The temperature was a very pleasant 72 degrees, with a good wind from the south. The clouds raced across the sky, and the steel roof started to make a lot of noise as the wind began to howl around the edges.

The next morning I found that a steel chair had flown from my porch, clear across the lawn, and landed in front of the cook shack. A small steel cabinet on my porch had been moved three feet and fallen over and the entire contents of a big box of large envelopes had flown off, only leaving behind the bottom of the box itself. The envelopes kept drifting ashore of the pond for days.

This change in the weather was followed by a full week of rain. When we again had a nice day, I watched the buds growing on a tree, hour by hour. By early March, the leaves were fully out.

If I had been living in a house, I would have thought of this winter as the mildest I had ever experienced, but with this semi-outdoor living, it was something else. The arrival of spring was eagerly awaited.

I still had my Ohio driver's license, though I had been in Texas for half a year. Sue had been there for a year, and Joanne also needed a new license. I had put it off, as it was an unpleasant hassle to go through, and I hardly drove anyway. Sue had found out that all the offices that could issue a new license were pesticided once a month, which made it impossible for her to go in there. She had then started asking for an accommodation of her disability, and finally it was accepted. We were visited by two nice ladies from the agency, who came out to the camp bringing a portable camera, eye tester and photographic background. The blue background was hung on the clothesline on my porch and our pictures were taken while one of the ladies held on to the bottom of the cloth, so it was steady in the wind.

The formalities were easy to get through, and soon we all three had our temporary driver's licenses. The two officers were very nice and had no trouble understanding what we were about.

They did house visits regularly for people with disabilities, typically people in nursing homes, who needed an ID card. When asked if this was the strangest place they had ever been, they replied that they had visited a yet more unusual place: an airtight domed building somewhere way north of Dallas, that housed some people with no immune system at all. The one officer who went inside had to go through a sterilization procedure first.

Joanne and I received our new licenses a month later, but Sue's did not arrive. When she finally called, she was told that it had been a procedural error to send the two officers out to us. They only do that for ID cards. The logic was that if we needed a driver's license, we could drive and thus drive ourselves to their office. Eventually, she did persuade them to release her license, after many phone calls.

20

Electric Summer

When the weather turned nice in early April, we started getting visitors on the weekends. People staying in Dr. Rea's condos came to check out country living, and some moved in a month later. We were starting to fill up.

I was very concerned about getting a new next-door neighbor in the duplex. Ellie was nice to steer people towards other vacant units, but she could not keep the one next to me empty and turn people away. I was hoping someone who was really electrically sensitive would show up, so I could have a safe neighbor. Renting both sides of the duplex was out of the question; the rent was expensive, and I was living off my savings.

An electrically sensitive guy from California came out to look at the room next door in early June. He had trouble tolerating the heat and would need the A/C to cool his room down in the afternoon while he was at the clinic, but he could not have it on when he was present. That would mean I could use my room in the morning and at night, but not in the afternoon. Not pleasant, but doable. Then he decided he liked another room better and moved in there.

Eventually someone moved into the room on the other side of the duplex. She agreed to keep the breakers off, even though she wasn't electrically sensitive. It didn't last long before the breakers were on again, and I would feel a burning sensation in my legs whenever I went inside my room. I had to sleep in my tent instead. Fortunately, she didn't stay long.

When my economy improved, I simply had to rent both sides of the duplex, even though I then spent more than two-thirds of my income on rent. I could not run the risk of someone else moving in, and perhaps staying when winter came.

The window air conditioner in the next-door room had not been run for years, and Ellie got it cleaned. She wanted it to blow itself clean and get a workout for a couple of hours. She warned me when she was about to turn it on, and I stepped about thirty feet away, which seemed like a safe distance. At least it was for the few other air conditioners in the camp that were in use.

This unit turned out to be a different model, more powerful. It was blowing me away at a thirty-foot distance! I was very uncomfortable, and got a totally new EMF symptom — my teeth felt like they had braces on. I had to be seventy feet away from it, and I became trapped on a little peninsula protruding out into the pond behind the building.

Ellie apparently forgot about it, and after a couple of hours, I really needed to go to the bathroom. I ignored the symptoms and walked up to the back of the building and threw the breakers to turn off the air conditioner from a distance of about fifteen feet — better than to have to walk into the room and turn it off, but I still took a big hit. Stupidly, I turned it back on again afterwards, instead of asking Ellie if it could be left off.

When I went to bed that night, my legs were still tingling, though I figured it would be gone by the morning. I had done my energy exercises extensively but had not quite been able to remove all the effects.

When I woke up the next morning, I felt totally wired up. I should have put up my tent and slept on the ground, which would have helped me discharge the effects during the night.

I got a taste of the new state of affairs the following night, after I went to bed in my room. It was dark and everything seemed fine; I was almost asleep. Then suddenly, like the flick of a switch, I could feel electrical currents running through me. I hoped it would just stop, but after about ten minutes of it, I got up to find out what caused it.

When I stepped outside, I could hear the roar of an air conditioner, about sixty feet away. I tried to walk over there but had to give up halfway across the lawn. The sensation of a current in my body was increasing and my teeth felt like they were in a painful vise grip. It would not have surprised me to see sparks flying off my teeth.

A friendly camp mate happened to walk by, and was kind to walk over and knock on the door and ask for the air conditioner to be turned down, and it was. I was surprised it was run so hard; it was only early June and it was not hot at night. The next morning I found out that the woman who slept there had problems sleeping because of her pains and was trying to numb herself with the cold.

When I got back inside my room, I felt so loaded with electrical charges that I put up my tent and slept on the ground for the night. I felt better the next morning, though there was still a humming sensation in my legs.

A camp mate who moved out in December had told me she had a lot of problems with the air conditioners during her five-year stay in the camp.

She eventually recovered enough to even use air-conditioning herself, but for three summers it was rough going.

To get away from the main camp, she had a small screened room built on a back lot, behind a little hill. She called it her oasis, and indeed it was. I wondered if I should start sleeping there myself. It was surrounded by trees and dense bushes on two sides and was close to an overgrown pond with stagnant water, so there would be a lot of mold. I hesitated, and then someone else needed it more.

At that time, we got a new camp mate, whom I shall refer to as Jack. He was one of those kind and gentle people one could wish were more common. He told me that he was just down for a couple of weeks to be checked out, then right back to work again, all fixed up. I must admit that I laughed at him. Nobody who needed to stay at the camp could be fixed up in a couple of weeks. He didn't like that too much, and unfortunately I was right.

During his first week, they did a SPECT brain scan on him. He had a strong reaction there, perhaps to the dye he was injected with. That same evening, he started having electrical sensitivities, where he had none before. He was so sensitive that it even astounded me, and I was one of the most sensitive I knew.

We also had a surgeon staying with us for a while. He could tell me some interesting things. One symptom I sometimes got from EMF exposures was that my left leg felt stiff. One time that was happening, he examined both my knees with his delicate surgeon fingers and concluded that the left definitely had a swelling under the kneecap. At least I do have one symptom that can be objectively verified — I had not told him which of my legs bothered me.

There was also a fellow whom we called Nevada Jack. He was as electrically sensitive as the other Jack and rarely ventured into the main part of the camp, except to use the bathroom in the morning when it was more electrically quiet. He stayed with us for two weeks, during which he camped on a little island out in the front lake that was accessible via a small causeway. Some evenings, I put up my tent out there for company.

He could only afford to go to the clinic for two weeks, before returning to Nevada, where he had spent the past six months living in the back of his truck. He usually parked his vehicle at night in little remote canyons on the north side of Lake Mead, near Las Vegas, where he had been living and his brother lived. He would then venture into Las Vegas now and then to pick up his mail and do laundry at his brother's apartment.

He had worked at a body shop for several years, spray painting trucks.

When the fumes made him too sick, he got a job repairing automatic doors at the many casinos, until he was too sick for that too. He tried other outdoor jobs, like washing windows, but had to give up. He fought with Social Security for years and had to declare bankruptcy, while having to live in his truck with basically no income other than what family and friends could spare.

While Nevada Jack was staying with us, I started having electrical symptoms for no apparent reason. I was now used to trouble on a daily basis with the air conditioners in the camp — it was impossible to fully avoid them — but I would be fine as long as I stayed out of their reach. But suddenly I was troubled no matter where I went. I took my bicycle and drove over to the forest preserve and sat there for hours. It was at least a mile from anything electrical, but I still had no peace. A cell phone tower had just been erected a mile from the camp, and another one a couple of miles away. They were sprouting up everywhere in those years, but I didn't think they could be the cause.

The federal prison in Seagoville had a lot of antennas on a big tower — could it be them doing something? Or the National Guard, which had a base behind the prison?

I asked Jack and Nevada Jack that evening, and they both had noticed mysterious symptoms as well.

The next two nights I slept in my tent next to Nevada Jack's truck out on the little island in the lake. I still felt wired in the morning, no matter what I did. In the afternoon, my symptoms got dramatically worse; I was getting worried. Meanwhile, the sky got darker, and by evening, it was clear that a storm was coming in. Around 9 P.M., we could see lightning in all directions, while it looked like the center of the storm would go right through Dallas, passing us to the west.

To my surprise, I felt better as the storm arrived. Both Jacks felt relief as well. I later learned that this was a major electrical storm that had come up from the Gulf of Mexico and caused a lot of damage in Houston, before heading further north. I have since experienced similar problems when big thunderstorms were approaching, then relief when they arrived. Perhaps they release the electrical tension in the air through their lightning.

In the middle of this storm, I was standing outside beside Nevada Jack while watching the Texas-size electrical storm roaring around us. We were both barefoot for better grounding, but we put our shoes on when we both could feel the lightning hitting the ground as gentle taps under our feet.

It took another day for my symptoms to simmer down to normal again, much to my relief.

As we got closer to July, the weather got hotter. The camp's air conditioners were used more, and turned on earlier in the day. My problems with them also got worse. Despite my efforts to stay away during the afternoons, I still got affected by them daily. It was impossible to avoid them completely. Where my principal occupation during the winter had been to stay warm, my primary concern for the rest of the summer was avoiding getting zapped by the air conditioners.

My biggest problem was a particular air conditioner, which was on the wall of a room directly across from mine. It was used by a young woman who refused to open any of her windows. When she had taken her morning shower, the air inside her room was saturated with moisture, which caused her clothes to become moldy — so much that some patients at the clinic complained that she smelled moldy. Instead of opening her windows to let the steam out, she used her air conditioner as a dehumidifier. This dramatically cut the time I had access to my own room to only a couple of hours very early in the morning. Debby tried to help me be in my room by suggesting I place a five-gallon glass bottle with saline in each corner of the room. This should absorb some of the EMF that was bouncing around between the steel walls. It helped a little, enough that I could tell the difference, but it was not enough.

I pleaded with the woman to consider my needs as well, some compromise, or at least tell me why it was important to keep her windows closed, but she was relentless and made me homeless for the summer. I was not able to sleep in my room for several months over the summer and far into the fall.

When it finally cooled down in the fall, everybody else stopped using their air conditioners, but she continued unabated. I couldn't figure out how she could even be in there — the room must have been like an ice box. Then someone told me that she was using an electric space heater in there too, an enormous waste of electricity. This went on for several more weeks, until she finally moved out, along with several other residents, to more comfortable winter quarters in Dr. Rea's apartments in Dallas.

During the summer, I would get up real early every morning before sunrise and pack my tent up to protect it from the sun during the day. Then I would have a few precious hours where I had the freedom to roam the camp. I would check for phone messages, take a shower, do paperwork and whatever else required access to my things. By mid-morning the air conditioners would start up and make the main part of the camp too uncomfortable and I would retreat for the day, usually sitting under a tree by the back pond or at the nearby park.

I wasn't doing well during the heat of the day anyway. I had done well with the heat the previous summer, but now it made me dizzy and I couldn't really do much. I had now been there a year and become allergic to everything in the air, which is probably what also made me less able to tolerate the heat. My head would feel like it was full of cotton balls, with my mind fuzzy and my vision blurry. I could not even concentrate enough to read anything — the words would just sort of pass through my head without registering. At the end of the page, I had forgotten what was on it.

It got so hot that it only took fifteen minutes for things from the freezer to fully thaw, and when someone left a case of bottled water out in the sun, the glass bottles exploded. One day I left my tent in the sun and it shrunk so it forever after was difficult to set up. I was working on offgassing a new tent, but it was slow going to make it usable. Modern tents are loaded with a toxic concoction of herbicides, mildewicides, flame retardants and plasticizers.

I spent many days just waiting for the sun to go down so it would cool off enough to clear my head. It was not a fun summer; I just had to let time pass until the weather would cool off, so I both could feel better and be free of the air conditioners. Of course, it could be worse. People could be toting cordless phones, cell phones and other gadgets around. At least wireless computers were not available yet. It did surprise me how few of the people in the camp had brought along a computer.

When Jack went back home in the fall, I moved into the oasis and slept there until it became too cold in December.

The oasis was a heaven to me in the warm dry fall. The mold levels were much lower than in the moist spring, and it was very quiet and secluded there. Jack had seen coyotes and even a bobcat one early morning. I didn't see any interesting animals, but there were a lot of microscopic critters that would climb into my bedding if I left it on the cot during the day. So every night, I had to carry all my bedding out there from my room, and back in again in the morning.

There were times over the summer that both Jack and I could sense electromagnetic radiation, without any visible cause. In late August we had a couple of weeks of it. Sometimes I would have unusual symptoms and even be bothered if I sat in a metal chair. We kept hoping for another big thunderstorm to come and remove what we thought might be the pre-storm tension in the air, like it had happened before, but none came. It was a problem regardless of where we were, whether in the camp, in Dallas or in the middle of the nature preserve. It did seem to ease off at night, however.

Then one of Debby's associates found the likely explanation: sun bursts. The sun sends out radiation across the electromagnetic spectrum, and the radiation varies over time. There is an eleven-year cycle of sun spots, and that summer was the peak of the cycle. It was so bad that communication satellites were knocked out and the northern lights were observed much farther south than normal. The November issue of *National Geographic* magazine even had a long article about it.

That explained what we were experiencing and why it was better at night, when the Earth itself shielded us from the sun's radiation. A website listed the solar radiation for each day and it seemed to correspond with what we experienced.

I didn't use the kitchen at all during the summer. It was extremely hot in there during the day, with the sun beating down on the metal roof. With a dozen refrigerators straining against the heat in the room next door, and a large electrical fan running in the kitchen, it was even worse.

The patio had a simple outdoor kitchen with a sink and a table, so I bought a portable two-burner stove and cooked outside all summer. That turned out to be delightful, except for the occasional rain shower. With so many people using the kitchen over the summer, there were a lot of conflicts in there, especially since some folks had a tendency to leave their dirty dishes in the sink, which attracted a truly amazing amount of ants. I didn't even walk through the kitchen door once for a whole month.

As all available rooms filled up over the summer, there were fourteen residents. The place was quite busy on evenings and weekends when the clinic was closed. With so many people together, people in an emotionally pressed situation, it was no wonder a lot of conflicts arose. Sometimes people would just feed off each other. There were especially many conflicts over sharing the six washing machines.

Many people arrived with clothes that were contaminated with fragrances, detergents and fabric softeners—either because they only recently were weaned off the toxic lifestyle, or because they had shared machines with other people.

The contaminants would leave a residue on the inside of the drum in the washers and dryers and then contaminate the clothes of the next user. A lot of heated arguments erupted over that. One person tried to solve the problem for herself by trying to hog one particular machine for her exclusive use. First she would clean it real nice inside, by rinsing it with peroxide and then run it multiple times without clothes in it. Then she would do a regular load, but leave the clothes in afterwards, so it was occupied for many hours. Other times, she would repeatedly run the machine with just a token load in it, like a sock or a single T-shirt. Ellie called her on it, and they very nearly ended up in a fist fight.

We tried to have a system where newcomers could only use two of the machines, while "cleaner" people used the other four, but some newcomers refused this system. I tried to stay out of these laundry wars. I only needed to wash once a week, and had the luxury of being there all the time, so I could watch who used the washers and choose one that had been used by a "safe" person. And I never used the clothes dryers during the summer. To me, it didn't make any sense to waste energy drying clothes, when the clothesline did such a good job in the Texas sun. But some people were even puzzled why I would use a clothesline, when a dryer was so much more convenient. I only had a couple loads of laundry get contaminated over the whole summer.

I have never been interested in gambling, but in that summer of financial distress, I did play the Texas Lottery a few times. Billboards along the freeways proclaimed that the winning pool topped a hundred million dollars several times, though that is of course a very misleading number. The actual value of a jackpot would be about half that. I have always thought lotteries to be a tax on poor people, who do not understand math, but it was fun to think about what I could do with serious money: I would create a foundation that would fund medical research and a program for medical students to specialize in environmental medicine, as none exist. I would also buy several square miles in the desert and build low-income housing for EIs and sell large lots for others to build safe houses on. The area would have very strict covenants to prohibit so many of society's problems, such as toxic laundry products, pesticides, fireplaces and cell phone towers.

I never won, but the experience made me better understand why poor people waste their scarce money on this pipe dream, as they have no other hope of getting out of their situation.

Since I stopped reading for several months, my over-the-top sensitivity to ink fumes had receded enough that I could handle reading a little again, very cautiously.

I offgassed a number of magazines and two books by moving them out into the sun every morning, opening them to a certain page. By noon, I would turn one page in each magazine and book, and take them all back in again by evening or if rain threatened. A lot of work, but I had little else to do and I was desperate for something to read.

It took all summer to offgas the two books. One book was *The Healthy House* by John Bower, about how to build houses that are less toxic. His wife has MCS, and their experience figuring it all out resulted in this book.

The book is a good start, though a lot of people I knew could not live in the houses he prescribed. The other book was *Hands of Light* by Barbara Brennan, which is about the type of healing work that Debby does.

I got hold of a medical study by Johns Hopkins, a prestigious research hospital in Baltimore. They had interviewed 4,000 randomly selected people in California about their health issues. There were some questions about chemical sensitivities, and 0.6 percent responded that they had to make major changes in their life to cope with everyday chemical exposures, while a whopping 16 percent reported being unusually sensitive to at least one chemical.

This was the first major study that showed that we were not alone, and it gave me hope that the medical community would soon start to take us seriously. How naive I was.

Other studies have later confirmed the study in California, but the authorities were no more interested.

My brother dug up a large report titled "Effects of Electromagnetic Fields on Molecules and Cells," which combined the results of 240 studies and concluded that human cells do get affected by very weak electromagnetic fields. It just could not say anything about whether there was any harm to it. Still, I took that as a vindication of sorts.

I have never seen any episodes of the TV series *Northern Exposure*, but a fan of the series told me that there were about seven episodes with a guy who had MCS and lived in a dome house, which he only left while wearing a space suit.

Ellie told me TV crews had visited the camp a few times but had acted very aggressively and made the people there look crazy to sensationalize things. She would no longer allow American TV crews on the property, but foreign crews were still welcome. I've never been impressed with American TV news, which tends to focus on entertaining rather than educating.

One day, a TV crew arrived from Germany. They had hoped to find a German patient, but there were none at the clinic at the moment. Since I speak some German, I was asked to participate. The journalist spoke excellent English, much better than my German, so we did it all in English anyway.

They took a lot of footage of the camp, with us walking around, sitting and talking, moving five-gallon water bottles around, etc. The next day, I went to the clinic for an appointment with Dr. Rea, and they asked to get me on film with Dr. Rea too. Afterwards, they filmed me shopping at Whole Foods together with another EI, both wearing our masks.

They first used a wireless microphone that bothered me in a strange way — it felt like someone was tapping with a finger on my left leg, just below the kneecap. I've never had that sensation before or since. They cheerfully plugged in a cord instead and that worked great.

They were really nice folks. They came from the German TV station ARD, their equivalent of PBS. They had promised to send a copy of the program, but it never arrived, though we know it aired in Europe as someone over there called Ellie to inquire about the camp.

Visiting physicians often spend a few days at Dr. Rea's clinic. Many of them are from other countries. They are often present during the consultations, just listening to the conversation. A few times, Dr. Rea introduced me as "one of his highly electrically sensitive patients" and asked if I would give the physician a quick rundown of my problems.

I was glad to see that outside physicians can show an interest, and they really did try to clean up for us, but it's hard to get it right. I tried to "live with it" a few times, but usually had to give up and Dr. Rea would then ask them to wait outside. When I apologized, he simply remarked that it is a good learning experience for the physician.

During one such incident, I waited too long to speak up. Once Dr. Rea got back to me, my mind was completely blank, and I had forgotten the list of questions I had in my hand. Dr. Rea just looked kindly at me because he could obviously see what was happening. The blankness passed in a moment, and we could continue. I'm always amazed that I remember those things so clearly.

Dr. Rea then told me that he himself had noticed an odor but could not identify it and figured one of his patients would. I sure did: it was fabric softener. I got a ride back to the camp right after that incident. We stopped at Whole Foods on the way to pick up a few things. I was still affected by the physician's fabric softener and had a splitting headache. My companion went to buy some fish, and when she came back, she found me staring vacantly at a row of olive oil bottles. It took hours to get out of that nasty reaction.

The destruction of the World Trade Center shocked everybody. The whole country must have been glued to their TV screens, but I had to wait until *Time* and *Newsweek* hit the newsstand to see pictures of it. I must be one of the very few people who have never watched the planes hit the skyscrapers on a TV screen.

The attack did not have much effect on my daily life. The effect was mostly that people seemed more nervous when I entered a store while wearing my mask. People started nervously asking me why I was wearing it. One person simply asked if I knew something she didn't — I was briefly tempted to tell her yes but then just shook my head. She just needed reassurance, not another complication to worry about.

I overheard Dr. Rea talk about a patient who had been en route to Dallas and was stranded in an airport for 48 hours. What a nightmare that would have been.

One day, we were no less than three passengers wearing masks while Lawrence drove us into Dallas from the camp. As we passed through downtown, a police car came up alongside of us while the officer took a real good look, but he did not pull us over.

Sometime later, I visited a large office supply store. The entire staff followed me around, keeping in contact with each other through the headsets they wore. Whenever I entered a new aisle, a staff member would be waiting for me, taking over from the one following me, in a sort of tag team. At checkout, the cashier nervously asked if I was a terrorist.

I do occasionally receive dumb remarks from people. Sometimes I ask them if they make fun of people in wheelchairs. Many people with severe MCS do not wear a mask. Some don't tolerate them, while others would rather be sick for a couple of days after shopping and keep their anonymity.

21

Camp Characters

We had a lot of people staying for a few weeks or months over the summer. All fourteen units in the camp were sometimes occupied. That made the camp much livelier than my first summer there, but also more difficult.

We decided to throw a party one Saturday. The excuse was the Kentucky Derby and that it was someone's birthday. We put up a small fourteen-inch TV outside and then we all watched the race at whatever distance we were comfortable. Some folks sat right at the TV. Three stood about thirty feet away, while two of us stood sixty feet away. At that distance, nothing could be seen, but it didn't matter.

It puzzled me for a long time that I needed to be that far away to be comfortable. Surely, the radiation should be gone around thirty feet or so. It was much later that I discovered that it was the electronic sound that was the problem. I could be closer to a TV that had the sound turned off, though not real close. Stereos and radios with a lower sound quality also bothered me more than systems with a better quality.

Sound sensitivity seems common among people with electrical sensitivity. I have heard about people who do better listening to books on tape that are read by a deep male voice, than a higher pitched female voice. Some musicians have also told me that there are certain sounds from certain instruments that really bother them.

We had a patient with severe food allergies. It was so bad that she could get blisters on the inside of her mouth. She got by eating really exotic foods, such as bear, beaver, tiger and kangaroo, that she got shipped from a company in Chicago. She was constantly experimenting with new foods and would interrupt any conversation to ask what a person was eating. Invariably she would declare that she could not eat that.

A humorous episode happened one day when she drove back from Dallas with another patient. They noticed a sign for ducks and rabbits and stopped to check it out. But the farmer really intended for his creatures to be family pets, not food on the table.

A few patients came to the clinic with such strong food allergies that they could not eat anything without severe symptoms. Sometimes, even mineral water would be a problem. They would usually look emaciated when they arrived.

A port was installed in their chest to bypass the digestive system, where the food reaction usually happened. Food and water were then slowly pumped into their blood stream through this port, using a little pump and a big glass bottle of liquid food.

It was not pleasant; they never stopped being hungry, but it worked. I saw them all slowly gain weight again, and after several months, their immune systems had "forgotten" enough about what it reacted so strongly to, that they could go back to eating normally.

Only a couple of patients every year had to go through that. One time it was even a child. It was extremely expensive and insurance companies often refused to pay for it.

One evening I sat with a camp mate. The woman had an asthmatic reaction and started wheezing. I had seen that before and wasn't concerned. One gets a bit callous about these things after a while. But then she went down on her knees and was wheezing very loudly. I just managed to grab her before she passed out and laid her on the floor. Then I realized that she had stopped breathing. It was dark and everybody else had retired for the evening. We did have a doctor staying with us at that time, but it was clear that the woman would be dead before I could get the doctor roused.

I had never done mouth-to-mouth, except on a dummy in the fifth grade, but I was it. I tried to breathe into her, but it just came out the nose. Okay, close the nose, try again. That worked better. Soon she started breathing on her own, but then stopped again. One more try. This time she continued breathing on her own and a few minutes later she woke up again. She had no feeling in her hands and legs, but an oxygen mask helped with that.

Many women stop getting their period when they get severe environmental illness. Some of them get it back after being on Dr. Rea's program for a while, a good sign of recovery. It would probably seem strange to an outsider that someone shares such news with the whole camp, but it was cause for celebration.

With so many people in the camp, we started to have some theft. The five-gallon bottles of spring water we stored in a separate building started to mysteriously become empty. Some people also had food stolen from their refrigerators.

The theft caused some people to buy water in one-liter glass bottles, which were not returnable. That generated a lot of trash as there was no recycling program. I couldn't stand to see so much waste, so I started to collect them, hoping I could persuade someone to bring them to a recycling dumpster. There were some dumpsters in progressive neighborhoods in Dallas, including one just a mile from Dr. Rea's clinic.

I did manage to convince one patient's mother to do one load, if I did the grunt work to load her car. That I did. I filled the car to the brim with well over two hundred bottles. The dear person actually did haul all of them to Dallas but told me that was the only trip she would do. She certainly had done her share.

We were briefly visited by a woman who had the most unusual reaction I had ever seen. If she were exposed to certain things, she would go into a catatonic seizure state, where she was unable to move a muscle. She would just sit there like a frozen statue. She was unable to speak, but her senses worked fine and she could understand what we said to her. After five minutes, she would be her normal self again.

It is easy to fixate on the people who continue to be sick, as the healthy ones do not need to come back, or at least rarely do. The year before, I had talked a few times with this cute young woman, who was very electrically sensitive. In the past year, she had all the mercury fillings removed from her teeth and that quickly made her 80 percent better, so she now looked the picture of health. I'd already had all the amalgams removed from my teeth, and it didn't seem to help me at all.

We had a woman staying with us for a week. She lived in a rural area and had to flee while a neighbor had his land sprayed from an airplane.

Another woman kept having problems tolerating her clothes, especially after some got contaminated in the shared washing machine. To get some relief, she would now and then go nude for most of a day. She then kept to herself and just sat on her porch, which was semi-private. This didn't bother any of us, though I really enjoyed watching Manuel nearly trip over his legs when he noticed her.

Then a young woman who stayed with us was visited by her parents one weekend. When her dad saw someone sit outside in the buff, he got so upset he went over to Ellie and demanded that everybody in the camp get tested for AIDS. Of course, he got nowhere with such a ridiculous demand.

Ellie told me that there was once a woman staying in the camp, who had such sensitive skin that she could not tolerate any clothes, but had to cover herself with bed sheets.

Another patient had stayed with us for some time, when she started to get severely electrically sensitive and had to stop driving her car. After being car-less for a month, she got so angry at her limitations that she decided to drive on willpower alone. She steeled herself and then drove her car all the way into Dallas. When she came back that evening, she looked terrible, but the next morning she did it again. That made her look like the living dead, and then she stopped this self-torture.

A new woman moved in over at Dolores's house in Seagoville. She came to visit the camp many times, especially when the neighbors were mowing their lawns. A doctor had given her high doses of a drug, which helped her greatly. She lived the normal toxic lifestyle for a while, until the drug stopped working. She was then worse than ever before and came to Dallas for help.

She couldn't afford much medical help and she kept getting worse and more desperate. Two years after she arrived, she bought a gun. Then she finally had peace.

22

Lab Work in New Orleans

To get more documentation for the appeal of my disability case, doctor Rea recommended I visit Dr. Rubin, an Ear-Nose-Throat specialist who had an extensive laboratory facility for testing the central nervous system. The problem was that he was located in New Orleans, about five hundred miles from Dallas. How to get there, and how to find a safe place to stay for the night, when I couldn't drive?

Going by airplane would be too scary, sealed up in a tin can for maybe two hours, with very little fresh air coming in and who knows how much EMF I would have to endure, with laptop computers, televisions and the airplane itself. I checked with Amtrak — yes, there is train service between Dallas and New Orleans, with a change of trains in San Antonio, Texas. It would take almost two days to get there, a very long time in a sealed-up passenger compartment with other people.

Greyhound buses get there in thirteen hours. Much better, but still a long haul sealed up with other people. It's mostly poor people who use buses, but even they have cell phones, and surely many of them will be heavy users of toxic fragrances.

I had some friends who lived in Natchitoches in northern Louisiana, halfway between Dallas and New Orleans. An overnight stay there could split the trip into two more manageable days, though it was still seven hours to Natchitoches from Dallas, with a bus change in Shreveport. And then five hours to New Orleans, with a change in Baton Rouge. I would still need to spend a night in New Orleans. The doctor said he would need me there for most of a day. There was nothing listed for the area in the *Safer Travel Directory*, and nobody I asked knew of any safe place to stay. Without a car, I could not stay at a campground.

Then I was able to talk Lawrence into the long trip. He really needed the money. I contacted Dr. Rubin in New Orleans and told him I was ready to come. Dr. Rubin replied that I had to get there the next day or the day after, or he could not see me for quite a while. Oops. Back to Lawrence, who agreed to leave the next morning. I faxed a note to Dr. Rubin that I was on the way.

The next day, Lawrence first showed up at noon to pick me up. While I was waiting for Lawrence, it occurred to me to call Dr. Rubin's office to make sure they knew I was coming. They transferred me to the doctor himself, who told me I had to be there at 6 A.M., without breakfast. Ouch, that's getting really tight now. It was the plan to stay the night in Natchitoches and then drive down to New Orleans early in the morning, but that early! Dr. Rubin helpfully suggested that if we left at 2 A.M., we could make it there by six.

I had to spring that one on Lawrence when he came to pick me up. We deferred the decision for later. Since he was doing the driving, I thought it was his choice anyway.

We stopped a couple of times for gas and to let me do a little grounding work. The many hours in the car did wear on me, even in the backseat. It was still much better than during the drive down from Ohio twelve months earlier.

We arrived in Natchitoches at four in the afternoon, and were warmly welcomed by my friends whom I knew from Dr. Rea's clinic. We lived next to each other for several weeks during my trip there in 1999.

They had a very nice two-story house with four bedrooms, a high-ceilinged living room and lots of open porches from which one can enjoy the peace and quiet of their five acres of forestland. It looked like heaven to me.

They had worked on making the house safer, and it was pretty good, except for the carpeting in most of the house. I could smell it a little, though it was several years old. They had recently installed a hardwood floor in one of the bedrooms, as a test before proceeding with the rest of the house.

We had a wonderful dinner, which happened to fully agree with the foods I had available on that day of my rotation diet. Much tastier fare, and a much nicer setting than in Seagoville, where most of us ate directly out of the pot. They had inquired about which foods I could not eat at all (such as corn and soy), but otherwise I had decided to give the meal plan a rest for a few days.

Lawrence preferred to drive on to New Orleans in the evening, rather than having to get up at 1:30 in the morning, so at eight we continued south on I-49.

We came through the city of Alexandria, which stank heavily of formaldehyde or something similar. Louisiana is a poor state, so the big chemical corporations have put a lot of their plants here where people are not able to complain much. They desperately need the jobs too. The stretch of the Mississippi River south of Baton Rouge is lined with them, giving it the nicknames "Chemical Corridor" and "Cancer Alley."

We took I-12 east from Baton Rouge, intending to stay at a state park just north of Lake Pontchartrain, and then crossing the lake on the bridge in the morning. In the town of Hammond there were signs for both a Quality Inn and a KOA campground. Staying there would shave off about half an hour's drive, as we could just zip down I-55 in the morning.

Lawrence had the experience that Quality Inns do not fragrance their rooms, so he wanted to try it. It was past midnight and the room was pretty good. I would have been tempted to stay there myself, if there had not been a lot of air-conditioners running in the other rooms. It was a hot and sticky night, no wonder they were all whirring away.

Lawrence dropped me off at the KOA campground nearby, where it was very quiet. I filled out the registration form and put up my tent at one of their three tent sites. No neighbors. Good place for the night, though not nice in the daytime, right next to the entrance driveway.

I got three hours of sleep before the alarm clock woke me up. I quickly packed up and was ready when Lawrence arrived at 4:40. It was tempting to take the registration form back again, the owner would never know, but I left it in the slot. An expensive three hours of rest: 50 dollars for Lawrence and 20 dollars for me.

I felt surprisingly rested, despite only sleeping three hours. Lawrence could not relax after all the driving and hardly got an hour's worth of sleep.

We drove down Interstate 55 and arrived a few minutes to six at the correct address.

The clinic was open, and I was quickly shown in to see Dr. Rubin.

I had some blood samples taken by a very deft lab technician and was then left to wait in another laboratory. After half an hour, another lab technician arrived and took me through a series of tests, where I had to wear some electrodes around my eyes.

The first test checked my sense of balance and was called posturography. I stepped inside a small booth, where the walls and the floor could move and tilt in all directions. I was subjected to increasingly complex combinations of these movements, including where the floor tilted in one direction, while the walls moved the other way. I was not able to keep my balance in the later tests, as I could not rely on vision to stand upright. The lab reports showed the movement of my head on a diagram, so it could be judged how well I responded to the challenges. Very slick.

The next "ride" was in a chair that slowly rotated in a darkened room.

On the back of the chair was mounted a laser, which projected a red dot on the wall in front of me. I was then to follow the laser dot with my eyes as the chair slowly turned. Somehow they measured how fast I could track it.

The third test was in another chair, where they put little bulbs of water into my ears, which changed the temperature in my inner ears. I then had to move my eyes between two points on the wall, while they changed the temperature.

Then I was put in a chair with a headphone on, which sent pulses of sound at various frequencies into my ear. I was not to do anything, but just to sit there passively. I was concerned about the EMF radiation from the headphones, as even a telephone bothers me, but it was quite manageable. My foot just got rather toasty, as a symptom.

Next was a hearing test inside a soundproof booth. First it was a series of tests where I should indicate which ear I heard a sound in, at various frequencies. Then the technician read aloud a series of words at a decreasing sound volume, and I should repeat each word back to her.

A technician affixed 32 electrodes on my head and then placed me in a soundproof room. There they recorded my brain waves, while I listened to music or a person speaking. They had assured me that the electrodes would not transmit anything to my brain, only listen to it. I did have an irresistible need to repeatedly blink my eyes, which I otherwise do not have a particular need for. This apparently did contaminate the measurements, but the person evaluating the data was able to compensate for it. I was told this was an advanced version of the regular EEG-type test, whatever that meant.

I was told to take a break and went outside to eat lunch. Lawrence sat outside and waited. He had driven back to the motel and tried to get some sleep but was not very successful. Check-out time was already at 11 A.M., so he rolled back to town and ate an ice cream while waiting.

The lab technician I had spent most of the morning with was outside smoking. I had not smelled any smoke on her, so she must have waited until we were done. I knew EIs were welcome here when I saw a sign on the entrance door asking people not to wear fragrances, and the clinic had an excellent indoor climate. It was only the waiting room and the bathroom that were not quite good enough. Remarkable. Perhaps Dr. Rubin is sensitive himself — that seems to be the common way to convince a physician.

The last item on the program was another meeting with Dr. Rubin. He already had a set of preliminary reports and told me they had found a number of problems, and that things correlated nicely as well, which should rule out that I was faking anything.

It sounded like the trip was well worth it, and we skipped town soon after. Lawrence was really tired, so we had to stop a few times along the way for him to rest. We arrived at my friends' house in Natchitoches just in time for dinner. Lawrence preferred to sleep in a motel instead of the house, so I gave him money to do that. He first tried a Motel 8 down the street, but it was very perfumey. His clothes stunk so bad he had to change them when he got back.

While Lawrence slept in the motel he finally found, I slept outside the house, well away from their air-conditioner. Fortunately, it was unseasonably cool for July and the air-conditioner rarely ran. It also helped that the house was heavily shaded by trees all day long.

The next morning I got a tour of Natchitoches, which is very charming with many wrought-iron balconies, like the French Quarter in New Orleans. Most of the houses were immaculate, with several converted to bed & breakfasts. The movie *Steel Magnolias* was filmed there. A very small farmers' market offered a little organic produce, otherwise one had to go to Shreveport or even farther away.

After another scrumptious lunch, we drove back towards Dallas. I knew we had crossed into Texas when I saw a Texas-shaped jacuzzi for sale along the freeway.

The lab reports looked impressive, with charts and diagrams. There were no explanations, so someone unfamiliar with them may not make much of it. I hoped they would impress someone. It was an expensive trip. In reality, it was a waste; the reports did not seem to impress the disability physicians. Most of them ignored the reports, probably not understanding them.

23

Stress Syndrome

Faith can move mountains, and fear can create them. Soldiers go off to war, experience horrible things, and come home different people with what used to be called "shell shock." Shell shock is now recognized by the medical community as Post Traumatic Stress Disorder (PTSD).

According to *Newsweek* (December 6, 2004), 30 percent of the soldiers who went to Vietnam suffer from PTSD, even decades after they returned.

Imagine yourself walking down a path. As you pass another person, he pulls out a long whip, gives you a good whack, and continues on as if nothing happened. You are momentarily stunned, and hurt, but the person is gone when you compose yourself. You continue on, passing other people without trouble, but suddenly the same thing happens again. Whack! This time you confront the person, who very defensively says he did no such thing. Yes, he carries a long whip, but so what, that is none of your business.

You spot a police officer and tell him the story. He flat out refuses to take you seriously and gets angry when you insist. You hurry home and tell your spouse, who tries to understand, but is a bit skeptical. It seems so bizarre, which you can only agree with. Except it did happen.

Your spouse agrees to walk along with you. You get whacked again, but each time your spouse just happens to look the other way. The painful whip lashings do not leave any marks, so you cannot prove it with anything. Your spouse tries to be supportive but eventually starts talking about finding a good psychologist.

You feel bad, your head hurts, you cannot think clearly, it is hard to know what to do. Naturally, you shy away from walking around any more, and from any other situation where you might get hurt. Or you may try to stay just an inch out of reach of anyone who might hurt you — and sometimes get too close — in order to not appear weird to other people. To try to act normal.

This is a taste of what it feels like to become stricken with MCS or electrical sensitivity. In real life it is much harder, as you are attacked from all sides at once, and frequently. And most of the people who attack are people you know, who you do not wish to offend by telling them that they really stink like a chemical factory.

At the same time, you are likely to be ridiculed, both by your friends, your family and by the authority figures, the doctors, who are not very helpful as Western medicine has a long history of treating people with suspicion instead of compassion, if the ailment is not well understood.

Friends and family may start to become distant and the patient may end up in more or less isolated captivity.

You learn that people cannot be trusted. The most common untruth is "I'm not wearing anything," when it is easy to smell that they are. Most people don't think of the fragrances that are in virtually all personal care and laundry products. They hardly notice it and do not intentionally lie. Sometimes people think, "Oh, it's only a little bit, we won't tell him and he'll be fine."

To an outside observer, it does seem odd that a person becomes agitated or fearful, or acts a little strange, when there seems to be no reason. The man who lathers on cologne in the morning hardly notices it, just like a smoker doesn't much notice his stench. How can that bother someone else? TV commercials have brainwashed people to think that it has to "smell clean," when clean really should not have a smell at all. Questioning that daily message will not be welcome many places either.

The patient often feels sick and unclear a lot of the time, perhaps all the time. Slowly watching while the good health, the job and the savings erode away is another stressor, which may be compounded if having to leave one's home, with no good place to go.

Sometimes we can add extra fuel to the fire ourselves. As my own ability to keep up with my demanding job diminished, I added more hours to my day in a self-destructive attempt to compensate. Of course, that meant I got less rest and probably sped up my eventual crash. It is well known that stress suppresses the immune system, so at the time we need it the most, the stress of the illness compounds the load on our bodies.

Professor Pamela Reed Gibson published in 1996 a study of 305 people with MCS to document the impact of MCS on people's daily lives. She has since published several articles on that subject.

It is extremely difficult to know where the limit of tolerance is, and that limit often changes during the day and with the season. It is dependent on how much the person has been exposed to that compound before and how much to other things recently.

With multiple exposures, we will also eventually become numbed to further insults—we can hardly tell good from bad any more. This is called "masking" and is what allows us to occasionally do some unhealthy things, like go shopping, and then deal with the fallout when we get home. It also makes truly scientific verification of both MCS and electrical sensitivity very difficult.

There are other factors that influence our tolerance level. One common one is that many of us can tolerate more if our blood sugar level is high, like right after a meal.

It is very hard to know at what distance something is safe enough right now, whether it is a fragranced person or a piece of electronics. And what is safe for two minutes may not be for ten. Do we know in advance how long we need to be there? That neighbor who just said hello, does she intend to just exchange a few pleasantries, or does she have something on her mind? Which way is the breeze going right now? How to get to stand upwind from this person without her noticing anything? Will she receive a call on her cell phone while next to me? Perhaps we can spend ten minutes in that store, perhaps not. If we cannot, the result may be burning sinuses for a couple of days, and a foggy mind for the rest of the day. Or even a sinus infection flaring up. Or a burning sensation for the rest of the day, from radiation.

People who are healthy simply do not have a reference to understand the profound personal impact this has. I used to be extremely healthy and remember not at all comprehending what it meant to have a bad back or any of the other problems I sometimes heard other people complain about, so I have seen the other side of this issue.

It is a stressor not feeling safe, not knowing when the next "hit" will be. To constantly have to gauge how close to get, how long to stay. To fake it, go along as if everything is fine. Having to discreetly change lanes at the checkout in a store because the lady wearing fabric softener just stepped in behind you. Or show interest in chemical foods you'd never eat, while you wait for the guy up ahead with the cell phone to move on. Constantly having to try if the ice is safe to tread on, and occasionally falling in.

This sort of life changes people, perhaps permanently. Just like our immune system is slightly altered every time it encounters a new virus, so are we all shaped by our life experiences.

It is no wonder there are a lot of "odd people" among the severe EIs. The important thing to note is that it is not specific to this illness at all, even to illnesses. To illustrate, I have looked at several personal accounts of stressful situations.

Journalist Terry Anderson was held hostage for seven years during the civil war in Lebanon. He describes the ordeal in his book *Den of Lions*. After a number of years, the emotional toll crops up in the story. He remarks that a psychiatrist would have a field day watching him and the three others he shared a room with. He talks about the hostilities they directed against each other, the petty territorialism, depressions, suspiciousness, withdrawal from each other and so on. One humorous example is his description of the exercising the four of them do walking around in a circle, one after the other. But, it absolutely had to be in a certain order. If one person was in the "wrong" place, it was not good. I can identify with him and the situation. Life in the camp showed these elements as well, though I am glad never to have been under armed guard.

Another interesting book is *Iranian Hostage* by Rocky Sickmann, who was held captive in the U.S. Embassy in Tehran for 444 days. He describes a nicer treatment by their captors than Terry Anderson, almost cordial. Still, he mentions many of the same types of psychological problems during the ordeal. He mentions two episodes of panic attacks after his release.

The book *Born on the Fourth of July* by Ron Kovic is about the author's life as a quadriplegic after being wounded in Vietnam. During his long hospital stay, he touches briefly on the behavior of the other patients, without much detail. He refers to the place as "it's a madhouse, it's a crazy house, it's a wild zoo, and we're the animals..."

When he gets out of the hospital, he enters into self-destructive behavior, like heavy drinking, senseless relationships and many prostitutes. He throws himself into anti-war protests and gets arrested, before sinking into depression. The book has also been made into a movie, which I have not seen.

I read two accounts of captivity in the Hanoi Hilton POW camp in Vietnam. *Scars and Stripes* by Captain Eugene B. McDaniel describes how some prisoners withdrew from the rest, while he himself seemed rather fixated on tapping messages on the walls, which was punishable by torture. There were also the usual problems of getting on each other's nerves, stealing food from each other and so on, though one gets the impression that the rituals of military discipline are good to hold on to.

In chapter 6 McDaniel stated: "it was the war inside — the battle against boredom, depression, anxiety, and the problem of just plain living together — that had its effect as well."

The diary of Anne Frank presents a famous story. She hid from the Nazis in a secluded apartment with five adults and two other teenagers. They were all in great health, but they could not leave the house and lived in constant fear of discovery.

She described many sorts of dysfunctional behavior, like the dentist she shares a bedroom with, and who refuses to let her use the table to do schoolwork — even just for two afternoons a week. And apparently, her parents did not try to resolve the issue. One wife also openly flirted with the other woman's husband, despite his open discouragements. At least what the young girl saw as that.

After six to twelve months, the situation took its toll on her: She could not sleep or eat, and she got depressed like everybody else there. It is clear that Anne was a very sensitive person. In her entry for Nov. 27, 1943, she mentioned a vision she had, seeing her friend Lies, who was captured by the Germans.

I recognize a lot of the personal behaviors described in these books from what I experienced living among so many EIs in the Seagoville camp. The anger, the suspicions, the depressions, anxieties, the hypervigilance and the withdrawal from other people. I saw a lot of odd behavior and some territorialism as well.

Is it appropriate to compare this "EI experience" with being held hostage or being in a POW camp? With being a wounded war veteran or a Jew in hiding? They are all extreme situations, with several elements in common — the confinement, the abuses and deprivations, the uncertainties, the constant pain. Of course, we were not under armed guard, but we were not free to leave either and there were other elements, such as feeling sick a lot of the time and the concern of being able to pay the high rent or face homelessness.

This book is not a scholarly work, just my attempt to tell a story and provide some perspective on a touchy issue, which is very much needed, as there are still people who try to write these illnesses off as just psychiatric problems so the rest of the world need pay no further notice.

Cancer surgeon Dr. Bernie Siegel writes about his experiences with the mind's ability to make us sick and well. In his book *Love, Medicine and Miracles*, he used several examples. He noticed that many of his cancer patients started to vomit when they arrived for their chemotherapy, even before they received it! They vomited simply because they expected to do it soon anyway.

He also described a study where a group of men were given a saline injection instead of chemotherapy. Thirty percent of the men lost their hair, simply because they expected it to happen.

The medical literature contains many articles about anxieties and other mental illness caused by traumatic stress, such as firestorms, earthquakes and other natural disasters, as well as car accidents, severe injury, concentration camps, hostage situations and other severe situations. They all show that a lot of people who go through these experiences get psychological disorders. I am not aware of studies looking at whether the symptoms of illness alone are enough to create a disorder, though.

In a study of World War II POWs, 28 percent of the soldiers still had PTSD forty years after the war, while 50 percent to 67 percent of them had it upon their release from captivity. Studies of patients hospitalized for burns show that about 29 percent have a disorder while hospitalized, while 22 percent did four months after discharge.

Anxiety and depression are also common among persons living with HIV/AIDS. A prevalence of nearly 50 percent is reported by one large American study.

The medical community is all too quick to label any illness they do not understand as having a mental origin. Probably because it is the most convenient, and it props up their arrogance — how many doctors will admit that they do not know? If the impact of the illness causes anxieties or other problems, it just reinforces the prejudice. In some cases, special interests actively support this prejudice.

The book *Asbestosis: Medical and Legal Aspects* by Barry Castleman describes the history of asbestosis. The health effects of working with asbestos were first noted in ancient Rome two thousand years ago, though it was not until the 1890s in Britain that the term asbestosis was first coined by a physician. North American asbestos manufacturers and one large insurance company, all well-known names today, fought to delay recognition of the illness. They funded research that showed no health effects and branded the sick workers as malingerers and mentally sick, which went on into the 1970s.

An article in the June 2005 issue of *Scientific American* quotes an industry executive: "Doubt is our product since it is the best means of competing with the 'body of fact' that exists in the mind of the general public." This was a tobacco executive, but such sentiment is hardly relegated to that industry alone, as the rest of the article bears out.

The January 2001 issue of the *Townsend Letter for Doctors and Patients* had several articles about MCS, including "Multiple Chemical Sensitivities Under Siege," by Dr. Ann McCampbell. According to this detailed article, the active efforts of the chemical industry to discredit the existence of MCS has been well underway since 1990. Using the same methods as the asbestos and tobacco industries, they have been successful in keeping the issue controversial by sponsoring various front organizations and producing biased research in much the same way as the Tobacco Institute.

The telecommunications industry appears to provide a similar bias. A study published in the January 2007 issue of *Environmental Health Perspectives* shows that only 33 percent of the telecom industry-funded research suggests any health effects from using a cell phone. Meanwhile, 71 percent to 82 percent of independently funded research does show effects.

Many members of the medical industry add to the problem by treating EIs with skepticism and sometimes outright hostility. They would rather blame the victim than admit to not understanding what the ailment is. In the past, sufferers of other syndromes, such as Lyme disease, multiple sclerosis, fibromyalgia, endometriosis, hyperacusis, chronic fatigue and even AIDS have been abused by medical professionals. Some still are.

It is important to realize that the field of psychiatry does not have many objective measurements to base a diagnosis on. It is the judgment of the physician, based on a set of criteria, that forms the diagnosis, not a test of the blood or urine, as it mostly is in other specialties.

When a person has physical symptoms without a generally accepted disease to explain it, it is likely to be considered a psychological disorder. This is especially so with more general symptoms, like pains in the head, dizziness and other common EI symptoms. When the patient also explains having problems in public places or handling certain items, the doctor will start thinking in terms of phobias. "Normal behavior" is a social norm, that depends on the local culture, not anything absolute. It is only recently that the diagnostic code for homosexuality as a psychological disorder was removed, for instance.

There have been a number of medical articles that look at psychological problems among people with environmental illness. The early ones mostly concluded that the illness itself is psychological.

One was published in the December 26, 1990, issue of the *Journal of the American Medical Association* and thus sent to all physicians in the U.S. It talks about a "subculture" that is "led" by "nontraditional practitioners" whose "treatments seemed to be limited only by the imagination." Then it continues on to disdainfully comment on the standard practice of converting a room in the home to be pollution free, as well as other measures that are quite reasonable when the illness is understood.

The fact that many of us associate with other people with the same illness is mentioned several times. Our general disregard for orthodox doctors also raises their eyebrows. Yes, surely, if one is critical of doctors, one really must be a little odd! And as for sticking to people with the same illness, it is a simple necessity to be safe and have a social life, as it is really hard to clean up a "normie," and keep them clean.

I doubt these psychiatrists consider membership in the local veterans organization any oddity, or perhaps the fact that people of many religious societies tend to stick together. Or what about monks and nuns? Or expatriate workers in foreign countries?

The article includes a study of 26 patients, recruited from a hospital and the author's own psychiatric clinic. The authors do express surprise that only two-thirds of the patients pass their criteria as having a mental disorder, though it does not alter their conclusion that MCS is purely a psychological problem.

Like most such early studies, they found that the sick people were mostly well-educated white middle-class women, which is probably taken as an indicator that it is all anxieties, though they do not explicitly state that.

The reality is that the illness is spread across all educational groups and financial classes, as later documented by larger population studies. The poorer and less educated people just do not have the ability to get past their primary physician, if they even have one, and take more charge of their own health.

It is true that about two-thirds of the MCS patients are women, but many illnesses are not gender balanced, such as autism, gout and Lou Gehrig's, which are all male-dominated. Women have a high incidence of auto-immune type diseases, like lupus and multiple sclerosis, which some doctors think may be related to MCS.

In a later article about the same 26 MCS patients, written by the same authors, they report that the patients show a high level of emotional stress on various tests—and they cannot see why that should be! Predictably, they quickly go on to conclude that this is caused by the psychological problems that the authors see as the foundation of all their ailments and all but accuse people with MCS of being hypochondriacs.

Eleven years later, the same primary author published a follow-up study of 18 of the original 26 people with MCS. All 26 were contacted, but eight refused to participate again — I would too, after reading the first article. The tone of this paper was at least more cordial than the first one. To the author's surprise, all of the 18 patients still considered themselves as having MCS and "remain resistant to psychological explanations of [their] illness." I must admit, I more think of someone else as being resistant to changing his mind.

Of course, not all papers forwarding the theory that MCS is a psychological disorder are like the ones just mentioned. The typical reasoning is that MCS does not have a proven disease mechanism and since it is possible to become sick by associating symptoms with certain smells or sights, it is reasonable to consider that. And it is.

A psychologist I met thought she had a psychological disorder herself before being diagnosed with MCS, and she spent years in the best therapy she could find — to no effect. Then she finally started looking elsewhere and eventually ended up in the Dallas clinic. Many have had to go through psychiatrists before finding an environmental doctor.

I have another friend who has no sense of smell at all — none — and has been like that since a child. She only has the basic food tastes (i.e., salty, sweet, etc.) and none of the nuances provided by the olfactory system. She reacts to "smells" just like the rest of us anyway. In fact, it is much worse, as she does not get the warning smells we get so she can move away from the problem before it makes her sick.

There are things that make me sick, even if I do not know they are there and I cannot smell, see or hear anything. Some things, like formaldehyde, make me sick at such low concentrations that I cannot smell them.

Of course, I sometimes do question myself — could it really be that I imagine these things? I think most of us wonder. But then I look at all the times I've been hurt by things I didn't know were there.

The fact that EIs tend to have emotional problems, like people in other stressful illnesses and situations, does not make the illness any less valid, just as cancer is not thought of as a psychological disorder, despite Dr. Siegel's anecdotes.

Studies have shown that there are significant psychological problems for many EIs, but that comes as a result of the illness. A study of 1,582 randomly selected people in Atlanta, Georgia, was published in the September 2003 issue of *Environmental Health Perspectives*. Like previous studies, it confirmed that about 13 percent of the population are bothered by chemicals to some degree, while a couple of percent had the MCS illness. Of those with MCS, only 1.4 percent reported emotional problems prior to becoming sick, while 37.7 percent had it afterwards, in this study. This matches the numbers for other serious experiences quite nicely.

The medical profession's treatment of vulnerable people is not just an observation of myself and fellow people with MCS. In her book *A Not Entirely Benign Procedure*, author Perri Klass describes her time in medical school and comments on the disdain the doctors bestow upon terminally ill patients — as if their dying is an insult to the doctor's professional pride.

Dr. Robert Krell published in 1990 an article about the psychiatric profession's treatment of Jewish Holocaust survivors. He quotes an earlier scholar on the question, "What can be the reason for their open or concealed hostility against those who have had to bear great sufferings?" which is answered with, "One major reason has to do with the contempt that man still tends to feel for the humiliated, for those who have had to submit to physical punishment, suffering and torture." In other words: blame the victim, a treatment many sexually assaulted women have been subjected to as well, when being seen by a physician afterwards.

For an account of how the medical profession deals with another emerging illness, the book *And the Band Played On* by Randy Shilts is a classic that chronicles the early years of the AIDS epidemic in the United States. Anyone who harbors notions about medicine being a noble profession can get them punctured here.

But it is not all doctors who fit into the mold of arrogant ignorance. There are still many who buck the trend of cookbook medicine and actually try to understand and help. Some more openly than others, though they may end up in trouble with their Medical Board. This book mentions some of these pioneers; I have met others who are not mentioned.

It is no wonder that the emotional problems that are common among the hardest-hit EIs are like the proverbial white elephant — everybody knows the problems are there but doesn't acknowledge them. It causes us to bristle at the suggestion of talking to a counselor, which is probably a good idea for most. It is routinely done for freed hostages and POWs. But, of course, nobody insults them by suggesting that what they had to go through was just in their mind.

The last subject to cover in this chapter is the fact that dysfunctional behavior is not always caused by emotional illness; it can also be a direct result of a physical illness. There is typically a lot of neurological damage in patients with MCS, which affects the body's ability to break down chemical substances, which instead accumulate in the body's fatty tissues, such as the brain. The neurological damage most commonly shows up as problems with short-term memory and concentration, sleep disturbances and inability to maintain balance while blindfolded. Obviously, other parts of the brain may be affected as well.

Dr. Theron Randolph already pointed out in the 1970s that reactions to foods and chemicals could cause profound changes in certain people. Pediatrician Dr. Doris Rapp has written several books about this and has published a video that vividly demonstrates these effects.

This has also been observed at Dr. Rea's clinic, which used to hospitalize people in a completely controlled environment. Already in the early 1980s, they published a paper that noted how the mental health of the patients would improve, simply from being in a safe environment and being free of pollution and only eating foods they were not allergic to.

This chapter mostly discussed MCS, but it also applies to electromagnetic hypersensitivity, EHS. EHS is a much newer phenomena, so there is much less data available. It is also an even less accepted ailment, so many of us with both MCS and EHS only mention MCS when we have to deal with orthodox physicians. Interestingly, the situation is the reverse in Sweden, where EHS is more accepted than MCS, perhaps thanks to a very well-organized patient organization there.

A list of references for this chapter appears as an appendix.

24

Trailer Dreams

Going through a winter in Seagoville, with hardly any warmth, and a summer dodging all the air conditioners, motivated me to find a better place to live. But how? The choices available were very limited for someone with severe chemical and electrosensitivities and no ability to drive.

During the summer, a new camp for people with MCS opened in the ranch country well outside Dallas. There was no housing available; instead, people had to bring their own trailers. Four people moved out there, and I became very interested. Maybe I could find a usable trailer and move there myself. I visited the camp a few times, but always felt "loaded" with electricity while there, though I couldn't see a reason for it.

I later learned about ground currents and inspected the wiring six years later, after the campground had been closed. The wiring was done in a way that could have created ground currents, but I could not tell for sure without the power connected to the wires. I had felt great there before any wiring was done and was still fine well outside the property.

Meanwhile, I had come up with a better idea where to put a trailer. The buildings at the Seagoville camp are located in a small section of the 48-acre property. Much of the rest consists of ponds and peninsulas left over from bygone gravel mining decades ago. There is also a fairly large island, connected to the community parking lot by a forty-foot causeway. It would be quite doable to put in an underground electrical line from the transformer on the side of the parking lot, and string a waterline from the main line that also goes through there.

Sewage was a problem, as I would be far from the septic tanks serving the rest of the property. It would not be possible to install a long pipe, and putting in a new septic tank would cost thousands of dollars. I was not willing to spend that much improving somebody else's property and the island was probably too small for the legal requirements anyway. I still hoped to be out of there within a few years, preferably less. With a trailer, I could later buy my own land and pay someone to move the trailer there, but that

178

still required reliable transportation, which I didn't have since I still could not drive myself.

The solution to the sewage problem came from an RV dealer. This problem is not limited to the EI world; other people also have the need to use a trailer in places with no hookups. RV dealers sell small sewage tanks on wheels that are placed under the trailer. When the holding tank is full, it is emptied into the sewage trailer by simply connecting the hoses. The sewage trailer is then pulled to a septic tank or dump station and emptied directly into it. I could do that with the septic tanks in the main part of the camp. I would connect the drains from the kitchen sink and the shower drain to a separate "gray-water" line, which would just go to a nearby hole filled with big rocks, so it would only be necessary to haul the "black" water. A weekly trip might be all that I would need to do.

I had been looking around for a trailer since late summer. I knew nothing about trailers. It seemed all I heard about was old Airstream trailers from the 1960s and 1970s, so I started looking for one. Some people told me it had to be a model from before 1969, when the company started to use plastic for the inner walls, and to avoid the International Series, where plastic was used even earlier. There were two old Airstreams at the camp though neither were used to house people anymore. One was an International Series, which always had an unpleasant smell to it, and only one person was ever able to live in it. Both trailers had been modified, with the inner surfaces covered with aluminum tape, and all the original woodwork removed. They were now only used for storage. At least these gave me an idea of what they were like.

Dallas is a wealthy city, with many RV dealers. One had a 26-foot Airstream from 1966 for sale. I sat inside the trailer for half an hour. It had a small sofa across the front end, with a kitchen area behind that. Further down was the bedroom with a narrow bed along one side and cabinets covering the other side of the aisle. The back of the cigar-shaped trailer was a tiny bathroom with a claustrophobic shower stall. Not much legroom in such a 26-foot trailer, but similar to what I was presently living in, though I would miss the nice windows. Both sides of the ceiling were lined with cabinets, and cabinets were tucked in everywhere in the cylinder-shaped space.

The trailer smelled strongly of wood, but I thought I would get used to it, or remove the cabinets. All the cabinetry was made of solid redwood, very nice. However, my mind started to glaze over after fifteen minutes. Perhaps there was mold in there; it was hard to smell it with all that wood smell, which could also simply be the smell of mold. When I got back to the car, Lawrence commented that I smelled moldy. The dealer told me they had replaced the floor in the bathroom, so there was probably some rotting going on below the floor. I was soon to learn that such work was a red flag for mold growth, and a very common one in old trailers.

I had brought along a Petri dish to test for mold, and when I got the report back, it showed a high level of mold and described the types of mold found and what surroundings they liked to be in.

I started buying a weekly magazine listing boats and RVs for sale, looking for older Airstreams and the copycat Avion trailers. Not many were available, and the couple I saw were not usable. One of them smelled heavily of Lysol disinfectant — wonder what they were trying to cover up...

Then I got in contact with two people who had refurbished old Airstreams for EIs. Both told me to forget about them, it was too much work. It is rare to find an old trailer that is not moldy, and the only way to get totally rid of it is to remove everything in the trailer, even the inner walls, which is an enormous job. The only advantage of the old Airstreams is that they are solidly built, the same way an airplane is built, and that the interior is composed of solid materials — aluminum walls and real wood cabinetry and flooring. Newer trailers are built with manufactured wood. They rarely last much beyond ten years, and it takes at least that amount of time for the formaldehyde to outgas. The weak areas are usually the roof and the plumbing, and once there is a leak, mold will follow and be nearly impossible to remove again. With the small airspace of such a trailer, it takes very little of an irritant to make the trailer uninhabitable.

I dumped the idea of finding a usable Airstream and started looking at newer models. Perhaps a well-built one that was 10–15 years old would work for me.

A few days before Christmas, I hired Lawrence to take me to three big RV dealers in Dallas. Two of them had only trailers that were 5–6 years old and still reeking of formaldehyde. The salesmen told me that there was no market for older trailers. The third stop was better.

The first salesperson smelled of cologne, so I asked for an unfragranced one. Being a customer does have that nice privilege! The second salesperson was very nice. I explained my needs, and he told me he had once had a customer with chemical sensitivity. That made things simpler. He first showed me some moldy trailers. It had rained a lot the last couple of days, and several of the trailers smelled quite musty. Little pools of water had collected on the dashboard of a couple motor homes. One bathroom had standing water on the floor. Lots of leaky roofs here.

Then he showed me a 34-foot Airstream fifth-wheel trailer from 1988.

It was in great condition and had lots of room inside, a nice upgrade from what I now had. It was cavernous compared to the cramped cigar-shaped Airstream trailers I had been looking at. I couldn't smell anything either, though my sinuses and my head in general were already messed up by all the trailers I had already entered that day.

I came back right before Christmas and sat inside the trailer for 2½ hours on a nice sunny day. Not bad. My mind did glaze over a bit after two hours, but there was some carpeting in there, and a lot of cabinetry that I could remove if I had to. I also noticed some tingling in my legs, which indicated EMF. There were power lines around the lot, but I also wondered if it could be a new mold symptom. I had noticed this tingling other places where there didn't seem to be any sources of electrical pollution. I did confirm much later that some mold could cause these symptoms and that mold actually made me more sensitive to EMF.

I came back a third time with a friend who had a lot of experience. He spent an hour looking it over in detail and found a soft spot by the front door. It turned out to continue into the storage space under the adjacent bathroom, where the floorboard was rotting. The salesperson got the shop manager to look at it, and he thought it would be a minor repair.

I was still concerned about the tingling I felt inside the trailer, and not as much outside it. I had observed this before, but not paid much attention to it. Metal structures do seem to make me more sensitive to EMF, but if I placed it in a pristine area, that should take care of that. Nothing is perfect, and this should only be for a few years, I hoped. The salesman offered to take the trailer over to a big open lot, away from any overhead power lines. We spent a couple of hours there, where I first did some grounding work outside and then sat inside the trailer. I still felt a light tingling all the time, even when I walked to a deserted area away from the trailer. Perhaps it was solar flares? I thought that was the reason, took a deep breath and bought the trailer. With taxes and all the rest, it came to about 14,000 dollars. It was only thanks to the back payments from the disability insurance that I could swing this one. A few days later, Debby could confirm that there had been extra high solar activity on that day.

It was a part of the deal that the RV dealer would fix the floor and then deliver the trailer to Seagoville. That gave me some days to cast the concrete pads for the four wheels of the trailer to rest upon, out on the little island. The groundskeeper, Manuel, is very good at this kind of work. I got busy clearing a path to the site through the tall grass, and then digging out the holes for the pads.

A week later, we were about to cast the concrete for the pads, when I got a phone call from the RV dealer. They had opened up the floor in the trailer, and found out that the rot was much more extensive than first thought. It would require 6,000 dollars to repair it, and there was mold everywhere underneath. The contract limited their work expense to 2,000 dollars, so they could have stuck me with the rest, and the trailer, which he knew would not work for me with all that mold in it. And fresh flooring that would take years to offgas. He told me he couldn't do that to me. A true gentleman.

Well, if there was one trailer, there should be more. But it was not that easy. Over the next months, I called all RV dealers within a hundred miles, and when they had something on their lot of the right kind, I would grill them on the condition of it, to avoid wasting an expensive trip. I now knew what to ask for, such as soft spots on the floor, discoloration on the ceiling, musty smells, any repair work, etc., etc. Several times I went to look at trailers, either hiring Lawrence or begging a ride off a neighbor. Sometimes I would ride in to Dr. Rea's clinic with a neighbor and then continue with Lawrence. We even went to Alvarado and Cleburne south of Fort Worth, and up to Denton.

There were a few trailers that seemed promising, including a huge one called King of the Road, but I didn't dare buy any of them. It was hard to gauge how much improvement I would be able to do on the indoor climate by removing the carpeting and working on the cabinets. Besides, I seemed to have this tingling sensation every time I went inside one of them. I observed that I had this tingling sensation when I went inside most of the rooms at the camp, regardless of whether the electrical breakers were on or off. It did vary from day to day, some days worse, some hardly anything. It seemed related to how well I was doing generally that day. It appeared that rooms with metal flooring were worse than those with tiled or concrete floors. Rooms with bigger windows also seemed better than those with small windows. The worst ones were the two Airstream trailers, with little windows and metal under the wooden floor on one, and metal floor on the other. My own room had metal flooring, which sometimes bothered me, especially if I walked on it with bare feet. However, three of the walls were mostly glass, and I usually did fine inside.

These observations made sense, as metal shields electromagnetic signals, or rather reflects them. Our bodies do emit electromagnetic signals, unbeknownst to most people. Excess energy is sent down into the ground via the feet, but if the floor is metal, it will be much harder to "connect" to the ground. For a person with severe disturbances in the body's energy system, that can cause problems.

The solution to the problem should then be to get a trailer made of fiberglass instead of aluminum. Even in those, there would be a lot of steel in the underlying frame, and the floor would be high off the ground, making contact with the ground more difficult, but it had to be investigated.

I called up some of the salespeople I had a good relationship with and asked for advice. They told me there were only a few fiberglass models made 10–15 years ago and gave me some models to look for. One was the Alfa line, and I was able to locate an older Alfa Grand Tourissimo on a lot south of Fort Worth. It was a 31-foot fifth-wheel trailer from 1989 in pretty good condition. I went and saw it, and it seemed like a good one, but I wanted to be sure. The boss entered the discussion and simply offered that I could spend a night there to find out. My new neighbor, Larry, volunteered to drive me over there, then Lawrence could drive me home the next day.

It was the first of April 2002, with nice weather after a couple of days of Texas-size rain showers. Larry drove me and stopped in the middle of a big parking lot, so I could do some grounding work before we got to the dealer. When we arrived at the dealership, the trailer smelled a bit musty from the humidity left by the rains. A good airing-out took care of that. There did not appear to be any leaks.

Larry wanted to be sure I could really stay the whole night, and it's good he did for it didn't work out with this trailer either. I returned back to Seagoville with him.

I went to see yet another well-built fiberglass trailer, a 1990 Hitchhiker, with the same result. A trailer didn't seem to be a viable solution to my housing problem, and I abandoned the search soon after. I just had to wait until I could find a house.

25

The Balmy Winter

With the mass exodus of people who moved to spend the winter in Dr. Rea's condos, I was suddenly the only person who used the cook shack. Ellie had her own kitchen and the three remaining camp mates never used the cook shack; they were rarely seen.

The camp was so quiet that Ellie and I invited a couple of people for Thanksgiving dinner. With one of our recluses, we were only five but had a nice dinner at a table we put up on the middle of the lawn.

We had about two dozen people move in and out over the summer, a circus that was suddenly replaced by a blessed peace. With all the air conditioners off, I was again able to freely roam the campus and to access my two rooms and my things any time I wanted to.

I still felt an unpleasant tingling sensation whenever I went inside my metal-clad rooms, even when nothing electrical was going on. Just the presence of the metal floor was apparently enough. I hoped it would get better, as I knew the Oasis that I slept in would not be suitable for the whole winter.

I continued sleeping in the Oasis into December, when the weather got cold, windy and rainy. By then, I had recovered enough from the summer's constant EMF exposures that my room was no longer a real problem. I could then only sense a light tingling in my feet if I stood on the metal floor in socks or bare feet. I felt fine when in bed, lifted a little off the floor.

Having the cook shack to myself was great. I used the opportunity to do some changes while I could do them unopposed. First I installed an electrical switch by the entrance door to control an outlet in the far end of the room. I twisted the wires, to limit the radiation from the long electrical cable, just like it is commonly done in computer networks and phone cables. This allowed me to use an electrical space heater, without having to go near it to turn it on and off. The following summer, the same remote control was used to operate a big fan in the kitchen.

I got hold of two timers, so two space heaters would turn themselves on at five in the morning and warm up the kitchen for me. One would turn itself off again at seven, while I turned the other one off when I entered the kitchen.

I had tried to insulate the cook shack with Reflectix over the summer but ran into a lot of resistance. Now I could put it up unhindered. What a difference! I now had a fairly warm place to spend a lot of time each day. It even stayed warm for hours after I turned the heater off. And there was nobody to cause trouble with burned or fried food or using the electrical ovens. It was a much more pleasant winter than the previous one.

I did not have any Christmas party to go to that year, but Ellie made a nice dinner for New Year's. It was cold and windy, so she served it in her own kitchen. She was nice to turn the breakers off, so I felt fine in there. We had two guests from Dolores's house, but they didn't feel well inside Ellie's kitchen, so they ate in their car and then left.

It had been two very bad years where very little went right. I hoped the new year would be better, and it was.

The winter was much milder than the first one there. It cooled down to the thirties most nights in January, but often warmed up into the sixties during the day. We did have one eighteen-degree night, but the only snow we ever got was a brief dusting in February.

When the temperature was forecast to go below 25 degrees, we had to keep the electrical heaters on in our rooms. Those nights I slept on the concrete floor of the recreation room and helped Ellie turn on the many heaters in the unoccupied rooms. I quickly figured out to use the breakers on the back of each building to do it, without getting close to the heater.

One cold night, two of the old heaters died and the pipes froze. One pipe burst so water dripped under the trailer when it thawed the next day.

I had been without the use of the phone for a full year, which was cumbersome and cut me off from the rest of the world. I had gotten by, checking my voice-mail every other day, as that could be done in a couple of minutes. It is amazing how brief people can be in the time it normally just takes to start a conversation, but the social protocol is different for voice mail.

One day I was sitting in the examination room, waiting for Dr. Rea. One of his stethoscopes was lying on the table. As I looked at it, it occurred to me that here was a device that transfers sound without electricity. Using an old phone I had picked up at a thrift store, I cut the handset in two pieces. Extending the wires to the lower part, I then had a handheld microphone. Then I took an eight-foot piece of Tygon oxygen tubing and attached it to the ear-piece from the handset, where the speaker is located. The other end of the tube I stuck in my ear. The sound simply traveled inside the tube to my ear, so I could put the speaker away from me. The speaker is driven by an electromagnet, which bothers me greatly when too close.

This setup worked right away. I had no symptoms at all, and could speak and hear freely. I used it cautiously the first week, then went ahead using it for hours at a time. It was a joy to hear the delighted surprise when I called up my parents.

I quickly received requests to convert other phones and made five within the next couple of months. Later, I found out that others had already had the same idea. There were even two people in Sweden who sold phones made by the same principle, though in a much nicer design and higher cost. I only charged for the materials for the conversion; my product was definitely not professionally designed and people who needed them were saddled with high expenses just to live.

One Swedish guy produced the "Slangofon" (which means "tube phone" in Swedish), which was an attachment with suction cups to put over a regular handset. The sound then traveled through tubes in both directions, with the user holding a special handset that was made of either plastic or wood. This design would work with any phone, even a pay-phone.

My phones were not a complete success. Some folks did not receive any relief, or only some relief. I myself had no trouble with it at all for over a year. Then I would have periods of weeks, or even months, where it would bother me. This would happen after a major exposure to EMF, that would make me more sensitive for awhile.

It was a shock to all of us when Dr. Rea had a heart attack in November and was flown to a hospital in Dallas from his ranch out by Lake Tawakoni. The clinic was kept running by another doctor, but we all knew that it could not survive without Dr. Rea. The mood at the clinic was very subdued for several weeks.

To everybody's relief, he pulled through and came back after a couple of months. He was asked many times whether he intended to retire soon. His reply was usually that he would stay until he was carried out of there. I believed it; he is one of the most dedicated people on Earth.

An engineer from an oil company came to stay with us for a week at the end of January.

He had drenching night sweats, like I used to have myself. He outgassed so much during the night, that Ellie had to wash the walls of his room with chlorine after he left.

I was glad for the company and rode into Dallas with him a few times. He struggled on for two more years in his job, until he could retire. Those two years laid a heavy toll on his health, but he had to do it.

Our groundskeeper, Manuel, was sick several times during the winter. He looked and sounded terrible, but he needed the money and showed up every day regardless. After a week, I gave him a handful of vitamin C tablets and a capsule of garlic oil. That worked like a miracle on him. Every time he got sick again, I gave him the same and it worked each time.

I used garlic myself to help on my ever-infected sinuses. The dry garlic that is in most garlic products had no effect, but raw garlic and garlic oil helped. In years past, I had used a lot of antibiotics, though they seemed no more effective and were likely to have been a major culprit in my food allergies.

I indulged in drinking a lot of hot teas in the cold season. I rotated them, but by spring they all bothered me anyway. Perhaps it was because of the mold that would grow on the leaves while they are being dried, similar to dried fruit. The cold season is always harder on my system. Some foods I tolerate better when it is warmer and I feel warmer myself.

The clothes I had brought with me from Ohio were being worn out. I bought a new pair of jeans, which turned out to be much harder to break in than a T-shirt. It took two months to get them usable. I washed them sixteen times, soaked them a couple of times, and otherwise let the weather beat on them on the clothesline. Later I learned that for several years all jeans come with their own built-in signature fragrance, each brand its own. They pioneered that idea.

The camp dog chased a kitten up in a tree one evening, making a loud racket. The poor kitten looked starved and alone, so I fed it some buffalo meat and let it sleep in the laundry room. The cat was obviously used to people, but nobody came to look for a lost kitten, so what to do? I love cats, but it would never work keeping it. The camp dog would eat it at her first opportunity, like she did any baby rabbit she caught.

Dolores just had to put their stray cat to sleep, but she didn't want a new one. Then the Mexican family that rented a trailer on the edge of the camp property came to pay their rent, and they gladly took it. It was just another pet with the dogs and cats they already had. I walked over to visit a couple of times and brought some cat food, but a week later the cat was killed by a pack of roving dogs.

I got a catalog from an Amish store in Ohio. Called Lehman's Non-Electric Catalog, it featured all sorts of household implements that were common a hundred years ago. I didn't order anything, but now I knew where to find a manual washing machine, a hand-cranked drill and many other non-electric tools of yesteryear. It was fun just to look at.

I had started offgassing magazines over the summer, by removing the staples and hanging each sheet up separately on the clothesline for a day. Then I would assemble them again and read them covered by a glass plate. Now I had a better idea what was going on in the world.

Sometimes the weekly magazines would have pages that were glued in. It was mostly advertising, that I could just tear out, but other times it would be articles too. I could not figure out why they would do that. I assumed the advertising would just appear in some parts of the country, but the articles should be the same everywhere. To offgas those, I had to hang them up with a lot of clothespins, so air could get to all the pages at the same time.

I experimented baking books in the oven in the kitchen, thinking the heat might better fuse the ink to the pages. The first experiment failed, with a burning book, but then I succeeded. The formula was to bake the books for 25 minutes at 250 degrees Fahrenheit. It only worked for ordinary books. Magazines, newspapers and books with slick paper did not work. It didn't improve moldy books either.

Baking the books stunk up the kitchen terribly, so I could only do it when nobody else was around. I could do a lot of books in a couple of hours, enough for many months, and it was great to be reading again after being virtually book-less for a year. I just needed to cover the open book with a glass plate, which was so much easier than the cumbersome and leaky cellophane bags that was my other option.

I didn't know if I would get more sensitized to the books again, so I spent my "reading allowance" more wisely this time and didn't read for entertainment for quite awhile. It took two years before I had to abandon this book-baking method.

I read *The Highly Sensitive Person* by Elaine Aron, which was a big "aha experience" for me. The author is a psychologist and highly sensitive herself. She describes the approximately twenty percent of the population who are highly sensitive in terms of temperament, and more in passing mentions that these same people also tend to have more health problems, especially allergies. She provides a very positive portrait of the typical sensitive person: strengths, weaknesses and behavior, which very nicely fit virtually every EI that I have ever met. The problem is just that our strengths are not so valued in the Western culture, which more celebrates the gung-ho cowboy type, even though these same personality types often rely on more introspective people for advice to avoid becoming too much the bull in the china closet. I think any EI ought to read this book, both for validation of who we are, and for better understanding the positive sides of it.

Another amazing book was *And the Band Played On* by Randy Shilts, which is a documentary story about the early years of the AIDS epidemic.

I had often wondered why the medical community was so boneheaded about MCS, even hostile. This book sheds a lot of light on the dark sides of modern medicine. We are certainly not the first group of people to present orthodox medicine with a problem that it is ill equipped to handle, and the response is quite the same. A few truly caring physicians go all out to help, while most of the profession holds back and are more interested in shoring up their own fiefdoms. There are many horror stories where greed and egotism get in the way of helping desperate people, culminating in a meeting between President Ronald Reagan and the French president François Mitterrand to settle who came first to discover the AIDS virus and thus get the Nobel Prize. The Pasteur Institute in Paris was apparently a year ahead of a very ambitious and well-connected researcher in America, but they got to share the Nobel Prize. A movie based on the book has also been produced, but I have never seen it.

I also read *The Body Electric* by Dr. Robert O. Becker, which is the story of his research on improving the healing of broken bones. He decided to start by looking at other species, which are much better at healing than humans. Through decades of experimentation he discovered that small electric currents can stimulate bone growth, and actually control it. It was complete heresy that electricity had any effect on the human body, besides electrical shocks, and he was ostracized by mainstream medical research to the point that he finally had to leave. Today, it is common practice to stimulate bone healing using electrical current. In a profession loaded with smart people with powerful egos, it is dangerous to pronounce the Earth round, when everybody thinks it's flat.

26

Disability Circus — Act 2

A lot of new documentation had accumulated over the summer, since the rejection of my disability application in the spring. Lawrence drove me to a doctor in New Orleans who produced a stack of impressive-looking reports, and then we did the "booth test."

The booth test took three days to do. Each morning I would arrive wearing my mask, to keep me feeling as well as possible, so I would have few symptoms. A medical assistant would then walk me to a room with a small glass booth, where I would spend several hours.

I first spent some time in the room to acclimatize myself, so we could record what symptoms I had prior to the test itself. During the test, the medical assistant would monitor my vital signs and administer a simple intelligence test a few times. The crucial part of the test was when a small dark glass bottle was placed on the floor in the glass booth. Neither the assistant nor myself knew what the bottle contained. On one day, it was a harmless saline solution; on the others, it was a minute dilution of formaldehyde, or ink. It was so diluted that it was completely odorless; I had no way of knowing what it was.

I had no problem with the saline solution, but the formaldehyde gave me trouble. I didn't know we were testing with formaldehyde. I thought we only tested the ink, so I was surprised that I had symptoms I normally do not get when exposed to printed materials. Besides the symptoms I could report, my blood pressure dropped for half an hour, while my pulse increased. There was no doubt.

Formaldehyde was one of their standard tests and they had measured the air in the booth to contain about 0.2 ppm (parts per million) of formaldehyde. A very low concentration. Formaldehyde is an important toxin to document, as it exists in so many things, such as paper products, glues, paints, building products, clothing and much more.

I now had supporting letters from a total of five physicians and a big stack of lab reports. I even put together two pages with ultra-brief biographies of these five doctors. It looked impressive — three of them were internationally known, including Dr. Rea himself, who had made more than 250 presentations in 16 countries and had his name on more than 120 medical papers.

Surely, this ought to impress the bureaucrats in Ohio. My case manager sure was impressed, though she told me that if I failed on the appeal, there was only a very slim chance to prevail later. She didn't know of anyone who had.

It had been expensive, but if that was what it took, it was worth it. If the secondary pension had not come through, I would not have been able to do it. Justice costs money and is thus not blind.

Doctors are slow writers, so all the time I could get, with extensions, was used. There was only a week left for the final deadline, when I mailed off the heavy envelope by certified mail.

The response came pretty fast — a summons to see a doctor in Ohio! When I called to complain, I was told it was a mistake; they would find one in the Dallas area. When I asked what type of doctor they were sending me to, they told me it was an allergist. I complained very strongly about the unfairness of being evaluated by a doctor who would be duty-bound to be biased against me. I was told they would consider it, but only their in-house physician could make such a decision. To their credit, they did send me to someone who understood what I was talking about.

His office did not smell of anything, but the carpeting seemed perhaps a bit moldy and I got dizzy after waiting there for fifteen minutes. I had to wait outside in the cold wind for a long time, before I was finally called in and shown into an examination room.

Dr. X entered the room and immediately started reading aloud a note he had received that instructed him to not perform any form of treatment and to terminate the session if we already knew each other. He then sat down and allowed me to speak freely for a couple of minutes and that was about all I was allowed to say for the next hour and a half we were together. I once read that American doctors allow patients to speak for an average of eighteen seconds before cutting them off, so I suppose I should be content with the two minutes I got in.

He informed me in his arrogant tone that MCS and electrical sensitivity are not accepted diagnoses and that he would only state in his report what he would be comfortable saying under oath in front of a judge. He would thus only be interested in what objective proof I could provide.

He went on and on, clearly relishing his captive audience. I knew very well the power this man had over me, so my main concern was not to do anything that would annoy or threaten the very fragile ego of this pompous man. I was not feeling well in his office, having not put on my mask, so I did not have the brain capacity to think of anything to interject, while trying to pay attention to his longwinded monologue. Most of what he said was quite irrelevant. He just liked to lecture, but once in awhile he would ask a question.

When I was asked, he would stop his stream of words to allow me a short answer of two or three words, before he would cut me off and continue with his drivel. I could not give an answer in a full sentence, no elaboration on anything.

I was glad to finally get out into the cold air and clear my head. Lawrence had been waiting for hours and was very bored. It was a lot of hours to pay him for sitting there, but at least he needed the money.

I was first allowed to see his report two months later. It was a very longwinded dictated letter. True to his promise, he said nothing controversial. The height of his support was to say that if I spoke the truth, I was certainly disabled, but since I could provide no proof, he could not support my case.

When I got hold of the report, Dr. Rea advised me to find a lawyer, but then a new summons landed in my mailbox. Now go see a Dr. Y. I sent Dr. Y a short letter, stating that I had environmental illness and had problems being in most offices. I requested that he mail me any questionnaire so I could fill it out ahead of time, to minimize my time in his office. This also indirectly prepared him a little for what my health problems were.

He replied back with a friendly note to explain that he did not use questionnaires and would not keep me there any longer than necessary.

Dr. Y had a small office in an ordinary office building in Dallas. He had no secretary and apparently only visited his spartan office for appointments. When I arrived, I found his door closed. I decided to go outside after waiting in the long corridor for a few minutes with my mask on. Every five to ten minutes, I put on my mask and went inside again to see if he had arrived. Still not there.

My presence had been noticed by people from other offices, who stood outside with their cigarettes. Surely, a man donning a mask to go inside must be a dangerous terrorist! This was about four months after the terror attack on the World Trade Center, so people were understandably a bit nervous, though I very much doubt any terrorist would act so obvious, or play mayhem on such an anonymous target.

Two security guards showed up, meaning business. They were skeptical of my story but were willing to use their cell phone to call Dr. Y's answering service. He called them back a few minutes later and told them that he did expect me and had actually forgotten the appointment but would be there shortly.

He arrived twenty minutes later and released me from the two guards, who had kept a very sharp watch over me meanwhile, even following me into the bathroom and being suspicious about the content of my water bottle. I took it good-naturedly; they were just doing their jobs in a time of hysteria and I found it rather humorous.

Dr. Y was apologetic and did not act like the common pompous doctor who can do nothing wrong. I liked him right away. The session was pleasant; he allowed me to talk freely and only asked a few intelligent questions now and then, while he watched me intently with his piercing eyes.

He then quietly told me that he had met someone like me before and would likely support me. That was such a relief! I just went home and awaited the outcome, not pursuing finding a lawyer in Ohio.

It only took a month, then I was notified that I was approved. It took them another three months to produce any money, but that was fine. Their health coverage kicked in right away, which was important. The report from Dr. Y was very supportive of my case. The only surprise was that he recommended that a detective be hired to verify that I really do use my mask when no doctor is watching. I had heard about detectives exposing frauds or trapping innocent people, but I wasn't really concerned. I did go into a few stores without my mask, accepting some discomfort in exchange for not having people stare at me. That could possibly have been used against me by a detective bent on entrapment.

I never noticed anybody observing me. Such a detective would have had a very boring and uncomfortable time watching me in the camp day after day. If done honestly, such a report could perhaps have been beneficial at later re-evaluations.

I did have to suffer the insult of being approved for disability, using a psychiatric diagnosis along the line of "He believes this so strongly that he indeed is sick." Since neither MCS nor electrical sensitivity are officially accepted ailments and do not have a diagnostic code under the ICD System (they do in a few European countries), very few people are awarded disability for the true cause. Some get it on other ailments, like Crohn's disease or multiple sclerosis or whatever else they suffer from, while the majority have to accept a psych label. Just one more indignity. Historically, people with other less-understood illnesses had to suffer through many years of being labeled psychiatric in some form or other, before the illness is accepted. Apparently, acceptance requires some sort of blood test in most cases.

I did entertain the idea of fighting on for an honest diagnosis but was strongly discouraged from doing that from all sides. So I left well enough alone.

27

The Third Summer

The year of 2002 was a time when things were looking up. My financial future was settled for the time being, and both the winter and the summer were more pleasant than the previous year. There were only a few residents in the camp over the summer and that made it so much more peaceful. There were no personality conflicts and only a few air conditioners were in use. The ACs that did run gave me no trouble, as long as I stayed about forty feet away, and that was easy enough. I slept in my room at night and had the freedom of movement at any time. I could even hike up and down the road outside the camp, without being bothered by the power line.

I now could go into Whole Foods without a respirator, and the cash registers no longer bothered me for the short time I was near them. Such an improvement from two years before, where I basically had to throw my credit card to the cashier, as I hastened through.

It was only on a few really hot nights that the ACs bothered me enough that I had to go sleep elsewhere. There was still the occasional day when I felt wired up, but it was not often. Then the air conditioners would bother me and I would feel an unpleasant tingling when I entered my steel room. A thunderstorm would then usually arrive the next day and relieve the tension in the air, so I had peace again. It was a time when I was finally allowed the peace to recover. I felt better and the constant headaches that had plagued me for years were no longer there all the time.

I tested my new boundaries in various ways. I borrowed a television with a built-in VCR and watched the movie *When Harry Met Sally*, which we had in the camp library. As the movie progressed, I had to move farther and farther away from the little twelve-inch TV. I managed to finish the movie, but paid for it with much increased sensitivities the next day. I didn't watch any more.

I experimented using my laptop computer. I set it up with long extension cords on the mouse and a keyboard, so I could sit back from the computer. I also placed my feet in a bucket of water to see if that helped. I was all right for about fifteen minutes, then it started bothering me and after around forty minutes I had to stop. I got so messed up I had to sleep in my tent that night, to be grounded all night long.

Debby worked on her patients in her own home that summer. It was a nice villa on the north side of Dallas, which she had renovated to be chemically safe with tiled floors, furniture made of natural materials and an extensive air handling system with filters and ultraviolet light. I always felt great there.

The house was near a Whole Foods store, so I usually combined visiting both of them. Lawrence would drop me off at Debby's for my appointment, and I would then walk to Whole Foods to shop before Lawrence picked me up again. Sometimes he would be quite late, so I would sit outside with my shopping cart for up to an hour. A few times people thought I was homeless and offered me money. One time, a person came out from the deli and offered me a free sandwich. I hope I never will need such charity, but it is nice to see that people will try to help.

We had some amusement at the camp when an armadillo dug a huge hole under Ellie's kitchen one night. These creatures are all armor and have an incredible ability to dig holes. Manuel wanted to take it home to cook it, so he tried to stick his arm down into the hole to pull it out. The armadillo didn't like that idea and delivered a sharp response. A neighbor then came over with a trap that he placed over the opening, but the creature was too smart and escaped.

We had a neighbor who liked to burn trash at night, usually after midnight. He probably assumed nobody would notice. I was awakened by it several times but could just put on my mask without really waking up and then go right back to sleep. Fortunately it wasn't that close.

The variety and size of the bugs in Texas never ceased to amaze me. They were simply a part of the landscape and usually caused no problem. One exception was the two bugs that chewed inch-long holes in the new pair of cotton shorts I was offgassing on the clothesline.

I once walked past the kitchen window while a camp mate was doing dishes. He squirted a little water at me through the window for the fun of it. Of course, I had to retaliate by getting the garden hose and spraying him back through the open window. He got a bit wet. I remarked that he should appreciate being hit with filtered water! Filtered? How? Well, it was sprayed through the insect screen on the window — a very coarse filter, but a filter nonetheless. He laughed a lot at that one. That's camp humor for ya.

There was also a couple who only stayed a week. The wife started to unmask to everything, now that they were away from their newly renovated house. Every evening I could see the pile of things thrown outside their room grow larger. They were not the typical type of people we normally saw, as they were working-class people who could obviously not afford to stay. Ellie commented that people without the money to get treatment and education would often just die slowly of things like kidney failure caused by untreated MCS. I think the husband knew it; he was heartbroken the evening before they drove home again.

A woman stayed with us for three weeks. She needed to have cataract surgery on one eye. She could not find a single eye surgeon who was willing to discuss the special concerns we with MCS have about surgery, anesthesia, etc., so she had to come to Dallas. She loved to hike and we hit it off right away. We went for walks around the area and hired Lawrence to drive us to downtown Dallas for Sunday hikes.

Downtown Dallas is deserted on weekends, so the air quality is good then. I had not visited it once in the two years I had now lived in Dallas, so we hiked around and looked at the buildings and plazas. We even went inside a palatial art museum with marble floors and walls and great air quality.

I was in the clinic testing room one day in May, getting tested for an allergy shot for grass smut (a sort of mold that grows on grass). I talked with a young mother who was there with her five-month-old baby. Both the mother and the baby had MCS. The baby's face was filled with red splotches. He was allergic to all the foods the poor mother tried to feed him, even her own breast milk and any kind of milk formula they could find.

Someone arranged three sing-along evenings in the courtyard at the clinic apartments. I managed to attend two of them, together with other people from the camp. It was quite cheerful, with a couple of patients who had brought their instruments, while about a dozen people joined in the singing.

A woman from Germany told me she was surprised that the big power line near Dr. Rea's clinic didn't bother her. They did back home, but not here. We figured it must be because the lines cycle 60 times a second in America, while it is 50 times a second in Europe. Research has suggested that some electrically sensitive people are only sensitive to certain frequencies. If she had stayed longer in America, she would probably get sensitive to 60 cycles as well.

I was glad to hear that there finally was a famous person who went public with having electrical sensitivity. The Director-General of the World Health Organization, Gro Harlem Brundtland, told the media that she could not be around cell phones or computers, shortly before she retired. I think the media in America completely ignored it, and it didn't receive much notice in Europe either, though she is very famous there for her good works and for being the Prime Minister of Norway for a decade. It took a famous Hollywood actor to get AIDS recognized in America; I guess we have to wait for some Hollywood celebrity to step forward — there are rumors of a few who quietly stepped out of the limelight because of MCS.

Dr. Brundtland was the head of the commission that introduced The Precautionary Principle, which is getting a lot of interest in Europe. This principle introduced new European laws that require chemical corporations to test new chemical compounds for their effects on humans, before they are marketed. Hitherto, it had been that the public acted as guinea pigs, and publicly funded research and grassroots organizations had to show a chemical is dangerous to eventually get it phased out — a protracted battle that often takes decades, if at all successful. The industry has been very successful in delaying the phase-out of mercury, lead, asbestos, cigarettes, several pesticides and many other things, at a huge cost to the public.

28

Wheels at Last

The weather was great at the end of April, with temperatures reaching into the eighties. I felt unusually well and wanted to test my limits. I had now been car-less for two years; it was time to try again. With my disability case finally settled, I now had money to actually try to solve this problem.

My own car was no longer street legal, but Ellie let me borrow her older Mazda pickup truck for a test run.

I took it around the block. Felt good, no problem. Then a larger circle. That was pretty good, just some stiffness in my knee and ankles. No burning sensations. I could live with that. I was elated; freedom seemed to be within reach suddenly. I continued on for an hour-long drive in the country. What a joy of freedom on a perfect day! I envisioned soon going on a house hunting trip to the desert — surely, in the mold-less climate out there, I would do even better.

I was doing fairly good when I returned, just stiff in the joints, which I was used to when exposed to EMF radiation. Still no burning. I got my gaussmeter out and measured the truck. It radiated about 3 milligauss by my feet, while my own car radiated 25 milligauss. Aha!

Then I started on my grounding exercises, to release the charge that had built up in my body and made the joints so stiff. The buildup was more than I had thought, and I was not able to release it, so I slept on the ground in my tent that night to help it along. I had clearly overloaded myself.

The next morning, I noticed that my electrical sensitivities were heightened and now as bad as the previous summer when I constantly got exposed in the camp. Air conditioners that hadn't bothered me this summer now suddenly did. I was getting concerned when it wasn't better the second day. The third day I was back to normal again, to my great relief.

I didn't drive the Mazda again, but I refused to give up. The Mazda was clearly better than my Acura; perhaps other models would be better yet. A few days later, Dolores came over with her friend, who drove a Ford truck. He let me measure it and it was also much lower than my car. Trucks seem to have the electrical wiring placed further from the driver, which helps.

A neighbor down the street had an older Ford truck. It was smaller, with a different body style, and measured as high as my own car.

I measured all vehicles I could get hold of, including Lawrence's car, which turned out to be the worst of them all — it measured a whopping 120 milligauss on the gas pedal, when the engine was revved up. But it was low enough for me to sit in the back.

I wasn't finding anything that was low enough, though. Then someone suggested I look at the old Volkswagen cars, which had the engine in the back. I knew the librarian in Seagoville drove one, so I biked down there and talked to her. Yes, she had a 1967 Volkswagen Beetle parked right outside. I was welcome to take a look. She told me its electrical system ran on 6 volts and was so weak that the headlights dimmed when the wipers ran. It was the lowest measured yet, only 1.7 milligauss. But not that much better. The problem was that the car is so small there really wasn't much distance to the engine in the rear, and the battery was located under the back seat, which was really close to the front seat in this tiny car. A lot of electricity was also routed through the ignition key. With extensive modifications of the wiring, I could lower the radiation, but probably not enough. I was also concerned about driving around in such a small car on roads dominated by ever-larger SUVs.

I had heard that some people used old diesel cars, which can run virtually without electricity. I didn't like the idea of a smoky diesel engine, but with caution, I might get away with it.

I got in contact with a guy who was already doing it, and got a lot of good suggestions from him. He recommended old Mercedes cars from before 1986.

I looked in the newspaper and the *Auto Trader* magazine, both listing several for sale. I called around to dealers, wondering if there were better deals on old Volvo or Volkswagen diesel cars. Even the Volvo dealer in Dallas suggested I only look at the old Mercedes cars, so I looked seriously at them.

I went out and looked at three suitable cars. The third one was a Mercedes 300SD from 1982 with about 150,000 miles on it. I had been assured by a mechanic that these cars were so well built that I could expect it to run 300,000 miles, perhaps as far as 500,000 miles.

I took it for a short test drive and did reasonably well, but it wasn't good enough. The owner seemed like an open-minded guy, so I told him what I needed the car for and whether he would accept that we did another test where a mechanic disconnected the alternator. He told me that he once had been very sick himself, and for about a week it seemed like electronic devices bothered him. He agreed to the test.

We met a few days later at a local mechanic, whom I had discussed the issue with. He disconnected the wire that energizes the electromagnet in the alternator and I took it for a twenty-minute spin. It didn't seem any better, so I was disappointed when I got back to them. The mechanic thought for a moment, then he disconnected the wire that carries current from the alternator to the battery. That made a big difference. The radiation level dropped from 1.8 milligauss to 0.4 milligauss. I took it out for another test drive. Definitely better, but it was not good when I took it down on the freeway.

To get any further, I would have to do more work on the car, which was not reasonable to do with three people waiting on me. I decided to go for it; there was no alternative than to make this expensive gamble.

There was a lot of work to do on the car. It smelled a bit of cologne, so I started by hiring Manuel to wash the interior several times with baking soda, vinegar and AFM SuperClean. I also ozoned it a few times, and generally let it sit with open windows in the sun. All this really helped.

I purchased a battery charger, as the alternator would never again be connected to the battery. The alternator had been permanently magnetized over the years, so it generated some EMF still, but a lot less than before. It could not be removed, as it was needed to tighten the belt for the water pump.

I went through each circuit, disconnecting the fuses for what was not absolutely necessary, such as the clock on the dashboard, the cruise control, the seat belt warning and so on.

I also measured how much each circuit consumed of electricity, so I had an idea what it took to run the car and what I would need of battery capacity. One circuit had a problem with a motor that operated one of the electrical windows. It consumed a whopping 160 watts all the time! When I measured that, I was holding the little multimeter in my hand. The jolt in the wire made my hand feel fuzzy, as if all the hairs stood up on it (they didn't). I spent a lot of effort checking through everything I could think of, but it really didn't make the car feel any better to me.

Then I ordered a set of shielding plates made of a special type of metal called mumetal. I installed several layers of them around the foot well, where the most radiation was. That helped. I could then drive in to Dallas on my own for the first time. That was a grand day. On the way back, it started to get painful, and the next couple of days I was more sensitive to the car and other things, so I did not repeat the trip.

Then I tried hiring the mechanic to wrap some of the shielding plates around the outside of the transmission, but it did not help and was removed again.

I was close, but couldn't seem to quite get there. I kept tinkering with it and gave up a few times, just to go out the next day and tinker with the darn thing again.

Then one day, I tried to start the engine and then completely disconnected the battery. The mechanic had assured me that the car could operate without any electricity at all, at least the engine and the transmission could. The dashboard was of course completely dead and the turn signals no longer worked, but it could drive just fine. I took it around the block, and still it bothered me! To my great surprise, the gaussmeter showed a reading close to my right leg, but only when the car was moving, and the reading got higher as I drove faster. How could that be?

I called the Mercedes dealer in Dallas and talked to one of their mechanics. He told me that the 300SD model had an electronic speedometer with a magnet inside the transmission that generated pulses, which are carried through a cable that went up the side of the center console. Right where I could measure the mysterious radiation. The other models did not have this feature.

Once again, I went to the local mechanic, who opened the back of the transmission and pulled out the magnet. That did it. I could now drive without discomfort. A few days later, I drove in to Dallas and back again with no problem.

Then I got bold and drove over to Fort Worth and went for a walk at the historic stockyards. I continued out to the country south of Fort Worth and ended up running the battery down, so someone had to jumpstart my car.

It was a trip of 5 or 6 hours all together. I did feel a little tingling and some stiffness in my joints coming back, but I was so used to that. This was working for me now.

With the magnet taken out of the transmission, I had no speedometer. I had tried to figure out another way to measure the speed, such as using a wind-speed indicator from an airplane, but driving without a speedometer turned out to be easy enough. I quickly learned to gauge the speed by watching the landscape and the other vehicles, and as long as cars were passing me now and then, I should be fine. I did not have the need to drive just above the speed limit.

I now had proof that this would work for me, so I spent the money to fix up the car. There were some repairs that were needed, and I installed a solar charging system. The solar panel was installed on the roof, using a roof rack that is usually intended for carrying bicycles and kayaks. For the casual observer, it just looked like an empty roof rack. A second battery was also installed in the trunk, and I was ready to go.

It had taken me two months to get the car working for me. It was now late August, so I needed to get going on my scouting trip. Operation Jailbreak was ready for the second phase.

29

Out of the Cage

I was ready to leave the morning of September 9, but it was raining. With the car's battery only charged by the solar panel, there would not be enough electricity to run the headlights. Someone checked the weather reports on the internet for Abilene, Amarillo and Albuquerque and I decided to wait a day.

It was cloudy the next morning, but I left at 9 A.M. and stopped at a rest area outside Abilene four hours later. I had been concerned whether I could stand the car well enough to drive for several hours every day and decided that if I could not reach Abilene on the first day, I would not be able to do the trip. I did great; I had no EMF symptoms at all. Leaving the Dallas area made me stronger.

I did have some problems with "fried dust," which bothered my sinuses. To heat the passenger compartment in the winter, an electronic valve sends hot water from the engine through a radiator in the dash board. When heat is not needed, the valve stays closed, which consumes electricity. As the voltage of the battery got lower during the cloudy day, the valve started to leak so the radiator heated up and with it the dust that had accumulated on it. It took me several days to figure that one out and put a clamp on the hose to block the hot water. When I got back to Dallas, I put a manual butterfly valve on the line and disconnected the electronic valve. This saved quite a bit of electricity and made the car better in cloudy weather.

I drove 250 miles on the first day and then set up camp around 5 P.M. at a park next to Lake Colorado. The campsite had electrical hookups, so the next morning I could use the battery charger to top off the batteries after cold-starting the engine. It takes a lot of electricity to start a cold diesel engine. When I later got the valve problem fixed, I no longer needed to use the battery charger during the long days of summer, and rarely in the winter.

On the second day, I continued up through the Texas panhandle and camped for the night in Palo Duro canyon near Amarillo. It had just started to rain and soon the roads were flooded for about an hour before the waters again receded. It was a bit early to stop, but the next possible place to camp was far away, and I couldn't drive in the rain without enough electricity to run the headlights. I had to be ever-mindful of keeping the solar-charged batteries happy and make absolutely sure I was safely in camp before sunset. It was also enjoyable to hike around the area a bit, once the rain stopped.

There were a lot of tent campers in the park and only one small bathhouse. I had to get up very early to take a shower before the hordes showed up with their fruity-fragranced shampoos.

I got an early start on this third day of travel and drove four hundred miles across New Mexico to Grants where I camped for the night at a campground. When I explained the special setup of my car, the owner cheerfully let me string a long extension cord to my campsite so I could charge the battery in my car.

The campground was located at 6500 feet elevation and it got cold at night. That was welcome, as the big air conditioner for the office building was only thirty feet from my tent. The air conditioner was running occasionally when I arrived, so I went for a walk until sunset. It then cooled down, and the air conditioner was silent all night.

I spent the next two days visiting an EI neighborhood outside Snowflake, Arizona. The first house was built in 1988 and since then several other people have built houses there. The altitude was nearly 6000 feet and seemed much cooler and windier than Dallas. But it was great to walk around without having to dodge fumes rolling in from the neighbors. And I felt great inside the houses I visited, although there were no houses available for rent.

I continued on to visit the Rimrock area south of Flagstaff, where I looked at three houses. The first one I really liked. I felt great inside and it had a very nice porch. But the neighbors were rather close and a new house was going up next door. I couldn't afford the rent anyway.

Then I looked at a straw bale house. It was very nice, but it smelled like a hay barn to me, which was probably the wheat boards used on the walls. It would not have worked for me.

The third house was a mobile home that two people were renovating, with the intent of renting out one of the bedrooms. The view was certainly excellent, but I didn't think the mobile home would work for me. I was especially concerned about the steel floor they were going to install, which turned out to be correct when I visited them again the following summer. The floor was then in place and it felt like walking on a vibrating surface.

In the town of Prescott Valley, next to Prescott, was an EI house built four years earlier. It had two tiny studio apartments on the side of the house to rent out, one of which was available. The rent was reasonable and the air quality perfect, but electrically I didn't feel so good in the entire area. It was like the trouble I had at Lake Tawakoni the year before, but not as bad. A couple of people have since told me that they too had mysterious symptoms in that area, perhaps ground currents or some sort of tension in the ground, as there is an earthquake fault line going through there. I thought I might be able to stay there for a shorter time, while scouting further around Arizona, but I never came back.

Then I visited a former camp mate from Seagoville. Her house was close to a busy power line, which bothered me. The lowest EMF reading in her house was 1 milligauss, too much for me, so we spent the afternoon together in the nearby park by Thumb Butte. To camp for the night, I just needed to drive a mile further behind Thumb Butte, where there were individual campsites along the Forest Service road.

The next day I headed up into Chino Valley and visited a smaller version of the Seagoville camp. There were only four units on ten acres of land. I didn't really know any of the six people living there, but I was welcome to visit. Being an EI opens many doors. It is like being a member of a secret society; we just need the secret handshake.

The place looked similar to the Seagoville camp, though each unit had its own little metal shed with a private kitchen. Two of the units were built by Dr. Lattieri, just like some of them in Seagoville.

I spent the night camping next to a house in Paulden. The owner was a woman named Misha, who had recently moved into her new house. It had been finished a year but had needed that time to air out, while she lived in a garden shed next to it, or slept in the back of her truck.

The house looked normal on the outside, with metal siding and a steel roof. Inside it was drywall with a plain concrete floor, as she could not afford tiling. The kitchen had no cabinetry, as wire-shelving was much cheaper than metal cabinets.

We ate dinner together shortly after sunset, and then watched the otherworldly spectacle of a rocket launch from Vandenberg Air Force Base in California, more than four hundred miles away. It was quite spectacular as the rocket and exhaust gases were illuminated by the sun behind the horizon.

Misha told me about a house she knew was available for rent in a little town named Meadview, at the west end of the Grand Canyon. She had a list of the materials used to build it, and it sounded good, so I decided to drive up there the next day. I knew there was a group of EIs living in nearby

Dolan Springs, including two I knew from Dallas, but I had first ruled out the place as too remote. With no really good prospects so far, I decided to give it a closer look.

I visited the two people in Dolan Springs and camped in their yard. They had gotten the key to the house in Meadview, which stood empty now. When we got there, it was clear I could not live in it. It was only 2½ years old and still smelled of fresh paint. Many of the less-toxic paints that are available still smell years later, and I do not do well with them. Otherwise it seemed like a good house. The owner had also built a shed in the yard to live in during the construction and initial offgassing of the house. The house was rented out three months later, to another EI who eventually bought it.

We toured the area around Meadview for the rest of the day, a very nice area with mountains, views and the blue Lake Mead impounded by Hoover Dam. Back in Dolan they showed me two houses that had been built by an investor. He had originally planned to build six houses, but the first two were not a success so no more were built. They were very nicely done, with many fancy details, but expensive and they also stank of paint. One of these houses was sold the next year; the other sat empty four more years.

Then they recalled that another EI in Dolan had just bought a house he was thinking of renovating and renting out, so we went over to visit him.

The house was still in need of a lot of work when I saw it. A new heating system was not installed yet, and the floor had to be redone with tiles. The bathroom also needed work. The place stank like furniture polish, but the house had only been open for two days after sitting empty for two years, so it was expected to smell. I later learned from the neighbor that the previous owner restored old furniture, which explained the smell. The house would be renovated to be safer for people with electrical sensitivity, by improving the electrical system and placing the heat pump and all the other electrical parts of the heating and cooling out in the garage, away from the main part of the house.

This house looked like it had a lot of potential for me, so I asked to be put on the waiting list for it. I was the first one; others later lined up behind me.

I spent three nights in Dolan and managed to get introduced to some of the local critters, including a rattlesnake, a scorpion, a tarantula and a black widow spider. It was mating season for the tarantulas, so they were scurrying around the patio after dark, giving me a good scare the first time one walked by my feet. They look horrific, but are not dangerous and actually can be curious about us. Some people have them as pets.

The house in Dolan was the last EI house I got to see on the trip. I didn't have good contacts in southern Arizona, and there wasn't anything for me to look at of interest. The rest of the trip was pretty much sightseeing and looking around to familiarize myself with areas that might be of interest, especially around Tucson.

As I was heading out of Tucson, I called up Chuck and Sherri, who I knew lived somewhere southeast of Tucson. I was told that their house was not safe at the moment because of what the neighbor was doing, so I was directed to a little hamlet called Rodeo on the Arizona–New Mexico state line. Here Sherri was camping in her small pop-up camper in the yard of some friends. It was a delightful couple who had recently moved from upstate New York and bought 120 acres to retire on. It was so pleasant that I stayed two nights before heading on to Dallas.

I briefly stopped in Las Cruces to visit Nancy, a now former colleague whom I last saw waving goodbye the day Don and I drove off from Columbus more than two years ago. She and her husband had meanwhile retired to the nicer climate of southern New Mexico.

As I was entering Fort Worth, just west of Dallas, I started to feel my car again. The minute electromagnetic emissions from the car had not bothered me at all since I left Dallas, but coming back to an area where I was sensitized to the pollen, mold and whatever, there was enough strain on my body to make me a little more sensitive to EMF. It was not a real problem, just some stiffness in my joints, just like before I left Dallas.

When I returned to the camp, I started to prepare for the move. My soon-to-be landlord wasn't sure when the house would be ready but thought it would be early in November. That was five or six weeks away and I hoped not to have to travel any later in the year.

It was clear that my car could not hold all my things any longer. I had acquired a modest amount of stuff during my stay in Seagoville, such as a mechanical typewriter, a vintage metal typewriter table and many books and various smaller things. I had arrived from Ohio with a carload of things; now I had two carloads.

I asked the mechanic if the car could pull a small trailer. He said it could — a small one, with emphasis on small. And small ones are really hard to find. He said he'd been looking for one himself for a couple of years. That wasn't encouraging, but I would try. The first place I went to look was at a trailer shop I had passed many times going into Dallas. I passed it a few times more, thinking that I really should have stopped, but somehow I didn't feel like it that day. A week later I did go in there.

It was a larger place with a workshop where they built their own trailers from scratch. Their models were displayed outside — horse trailers, trailers to haul heavy machinery and some smaller ones, but all way too big for me. The owner came out, a tall friendly Texan with Stetson hat and accent to match. He had actually worked as a real cowboy in his younger days. Well, yes, they actually have such an itty-bitty thing out back that someone had sold them as a trade-in! It was the perfect thing, a home-built trailer that was only six feet long with a sturdy wooden crate on top. They had only gotten it a day or two before and it only cost what U-Haul would have charged for renting me their smallest trailer.

If I had gone to this store the two other times I could have done it, I would have missed this trailer. And if I had come a few days later, it would probably have been sold already. To top it off, it had an Arizona license plate on it. Surely a good omen for the upcoming move.

A few days later, I got a pull knob installed on the back of my car, and I was pretty much ready to go.

30

Fall 2002

I could really tell the difference coming back to Dallas again. Certain foods again gave me a stomachache, my head was again clogged up and my electrical sensitivities took a step up again. In Arizona, I could use a pay-phone for about twenty minutes, while it would be too painful after just a minute or two in Dallas. The humid air in Texas also seemed to carry more fragrances and other pollution from people.

It didn't help that we got an early fall that year, with a rainy and cool October. But I didn't care; I had a ticket out now.

I had left on my scouting trip as soon as the car was ready, and I had hardly been anywhere in the Dallas area. While waiting for the go-ahead to move, I did some trips, while being careful not to overdo the exposures.

The Sierra Club has outings open to the public and I went on one of them in an area near Joe Pool Lake. Two dozen people went on this hike, who were delightful to talk to along the way. People just like myself before my life was changed. I made sure never to talk about my illness; I wanted it to be a "normal" day. When people asked what I did for a living, I just told them I was a computer engineer, but just not working at the moment. Of course, it was not possible to make it all normal, as several people wore scented sunscreen and I sadly had to decline when there was lunch at a restaurant afterwards.

A friend from Ohio came down with his family to visit someone in Dallas, and they all came out to visit me for an afternoon. That was nice. It was they who had treated me to a pizza shortly before I left Ohio. His wife was now pregnant with their second child.

My parents live overseas and came for a long-planned visit. They had wanted to visit me in Seagoville earlier, but I didn't want them to see how sick I was then. Now turned out to be the perfect time.

Since I was moving to "the end of the world," I made sure to stock up on things that might be hard to get out there, such as books from the ware-house-sized Half Price Books flagship store in Dallas.

The Sunday before Thanksgiving was a nice sunny day and I drove downtown to go for a walk. The square in front of town hall was full of tables where a church served Thanksgiving dinner for all the homeless people there. There were at least a couple hundred of these unfortunate souls.

I could have ended up there myself. Most EIs that are homeless live in their cars, but since I couldn't drive, that would not work for long as homeless people are always chased away. And using a shelter for the homeless would be completely impossible. I wonder if any of those people I saw were EI, perhaps without knowing it. Most homeless people are sick in some way.

A university in Philadelphia awarded their Man of the Year prize to Dr. Rea for his "contribution to mankind." That was nice; he has had to endure a lot of backbiting from the medical establishment for being a pioneer, though I don't think he was forced out from anywhere for his heretical thinking. That did happen to Dr. Theron Randolph, who was Dr. Rea's mentor.

The camp was still lightly inhabited during the fall. Besides Ellie and the two reclusive permanent inmates, there was just a married couple and myself. The husband went to watch the game at a sports bar one time and headed directly into the shower when he came back. She probably made him strip outside, but I never asked. I could smell smoke coming out of the pores of his skin for the next two days, even six feet away.

The West Nile Virus arrived in Dallas and they started aerial spraying for the mosquitoes in the northern suburbs of Dallas. It was our luck that they do not spray in areas where poor people live, even though with all the wetlands around us, we probably supplied all of Dallas with mosquitoes. They were plentiful enough right after sunset. One woman from the sprayed areas rented a room in the camp to sleep in at night, while she spent her day at home. She would arrive after dark and leave early in the morning. I never got to meet her.

31

The Move

It took longer than expected to get the house in Arizona ready. There were problems with the contractors not showing up and not doing quality work. The tiled floor had to be torn up and be redone and finally the third contractor finished the job. The new heating ducts and heat pump had to be aired out, which took a month, running it around the clock at a high temperature.

Finally, in December, I got the go-ahead to come. It was then raining briskly in Dallas and I had to delay the departure for two days before it cleared up. I conferred twice with the local weather service, which first wanted to know why I needed the information before they would talk to me. The first time, I just vaguely told them that I had a transport that didn't like rain, instead of trying to explain the whole thing. The second time, I told them that I was driving a solar-powered car, which was accepted without any comment.

The first day went very well; I made it all the way to Monahans State Park, 400 miles west of Dallas. It was cloudy most of the way and the batteries were in need of a charge when I arrived at 4:30 P.M. with very little daylight left.

There were only a couple RVs camped in the park, all nice and quiet. The park's restrooms were heated with vent-less propane heaters, which made them totally unusable to me. The theory with these heaters is that they burn so cleanly that there is no need for a chimney, but that is just a theory. It was so bad in there that my respirator was no help at all.

It was a chilly 38 degrees the next morning, but I was well equipped for it. I woke up well before sunrise and walked around until the sun rose over the sand dunes, so I could leave. The camp site had an electrical outlet, so I could roll out of there with fully charged batteries, after a very cold start.

I stopped at a Wendy's in the town of Monahans to use their bathroom and had to park in the space designated for trucks, as the trailer would not fit a regular space. My car and the itty-bitty trailer looked really diminutive next to the eighteen-wheelers.

It was still morning when I passed over the very southern end of the Rockies. They are only low hills there, but enough to be shrouded in fog that morning. I ran the parking lights on the car to conserve energy and hoped no cop would see me. The main thing was the tail lights anyway, and the traffic was very light.

It was again a cloudy day, and this time of the year the sun never gets high in the sky so it never bears directly down on the solar panel on the roof. In the warmer season there would be little concern about how the batteries were doing, but on this December day I kept glancing at the slowly sinking voltmeter dial as I passed through El Paso and headed west through New Mexico.

I stopped in Deming to fill the tank. I told the station owner that my battery was weak and he let me give it a fifteen-minute boost with the battery charger. I didn't have time for more, as the day was waning, but it helped so I could make it all the way to those nice folks in Rodeo, New Mexico. I made it, just as the sun went down. A bit reckless, but much nicer than any campground around Deming.

I had made very good time on this trip. The third day was more leisurely, as I only needed to make it to Picacho Peak State Park south of Phoenix. It was the last campground before Phoenix, and for quite a distance after. It was at a lower elevation and while there was frost on my tent in the morning in Rodeo, I could hike around the park almost in a T-shirt in the late afternoon.

I had scouted out a restroom that was away from all the campers, so I could get a comfortable shower in the evening, without having to sniff other people's toiletries. And the next morning I parked the car right in front of the entrance and strung a long electrical cord inside to top off the batteries before I left on the final leg in the clear sunshine.

Driving through Phoenix with the little trailer was unpleasant, as people there are even worse drivers than in Dallas. I had chosen the route through Wickenburg because it was the fastest and the least hilly. The car had trouble getting hot climbing up some of the long hills, pulling the trailer, which meant trailing a line of cars behind on the two-lane sections of the highway. Irritated drivers made sure to let me know their displeasure.

It was mid-afternoon when I reached Dolan Springs and I was met at the house by my landlord. I had rented it for a week to try it out first. With the problems I had, I rented it a week at a time, until I could sign a lease contract at New Year's.

First thing to make it habitable was to move the refrigerator out in the garage, so the noise and radiation wouldn't bother me. There was a smell of fresh concrete from the tile grout, but it seemed O.K. However, I was very groggy when I woke up the next morning. The second night, I slept in another place but had the same grogginess. Some of the local EIs came over to sniff out the place and lend me their opinions— some liked the front bedroom, some the rear one, and so on. One person lent me some non-toxic grout sealer (mostly sodium silicate) so I could get started, while another one came with some "Tu-Tuff" material to cover the floor with.

I camped outside while working on the house and first tried to sleep inside several days later. Neither of the bedrooms worked for me, so I ended up in the living room.

The bathroom was the only room that had been heavily renovated and still smelled of the paint and caulking, but I kept the window open all the time and after a year the smells were no longer noticeable.

The heat pump did bother me some, so I used it sparingly, usually when I was away from the house. Initially, I used a low–EMF electric space heater, which I kept well away from me, but after several weeks, it bothered me too much. I was used to very poorly heated rooms from the camp, so this was still a big step up with this much heat. It was also an adjustment for my sinuses to live in the super-dry air inside the house.

There were no pine trees in Dolan, but I had brought a string of lights that I hung over a Joshua Tree, which looked really nice. On Christmas Day I went to a nice party at a house in nearby Meadview, where I got to meet more of the local EIs. There were two out-of-town visitors too, whom I happened to know already.

One was Nevada Jack, who stayed briefly in Seagoville the year before, and was still living in the back of his truck outside Las Vegas.

The woman who hosted the Christmas party committed suicide two years later.

32

Desert Exile

Dolan Springs was a world apart. It was a place where one could buy a modest home on a one-acre lot with mountain views, and only pay about $30,000 for it. But it was far away from everything.

It was a place that had attracted a lot of people on a modest income: a lot of retired blue-collar workers, people with various disabilities and people who just wanted to be left alone.

I heard the story that until recently, when a prisoner was released from a prison in Phoenix, he would be offered a free one-way Greyhound ticket to Kingman — the last frontier of Arizona.

Dolan was a place where one could bring in an old travel trailer to live in and then slowly build a house around it with whatever one could scrounge for materials. There were no building inspectors; they would first start coming up there in 2007.

About fifteen hundred people lived in Dolan and the surrounding area. The downtown was a dusty desert town, with a two-lane country road going through it, the one paved road in the area. The nearest traffic light was in Kingman, thirty-five miles away. The town was so small that people sometimes only specified the last four digits of their phone number. Every number in the valley started with (928)-767.

There was a grocery store, a small library, a bank, a number of tiny rustic shops that came and went, and four bars. The bars were doing well; not much else to do there.

There were also five churches, which all kept a respectful distance from Dolan. One was a fundamentalist church down the street from me. It had been painted pink because of a mistake, but now everybody simply called it the Pink Church and they kept the color.

I lived near the school, which sat on a slope, high above town. They got a new security system installed one year, which included a public announcement system to be used in emergencies. It had speakers everywhere inside the school, as well as on the outside. The staff quickly found out that this system was handy for calling people to the phone, so a dozen times a day, all classrooms and the valley below were informed when John had a call on line three. It took a year, and a new principal, to get that stopped.

The typical Dolanite was past his prime, chain smoked and often cheerfully ignorant of even the most basic things, in the way people are when all their learning comes from watching popular television.

There were of course exceptions. The little library had an active group of supporters, which held book sales and other activities, for example. The only non–EI friend I ever had was a retired miner, who lived up in the hills a mile from my house, at the end of a road even UPS refused to traverse. He had no electricity, no refrigerator and heated his rustic house with kerosene. He was reclusive but well read, so we could have wide-ranging discussions when I hiked over there.

Another non–EI I enjoyed talking to was a local mechanic, who had a little shop. He just enjoyed puttering around with older cars, with lots of friends stopping by to hang out. One of his hobbies was building desert buggies; little two-seat vehicles made of steel pipes, four wheels and a vintage Volkswagen engine hanging out the back. An old beer keg as gas tank, no windshield, doors or lights. He knew how to live.

There were very few young people. They tended to run off as soon as they could, as there were no opportunities for jobs. The military was a common way to get out, and this little town had no less than three veterans' organizations.

At the elections, the town only grudgingly went to the Democrats, though Mohave County always went to the Republicans—so much that there rarely were Democratic candidates for local offices.

Drunk drivers were a problem. One evening one of them took down an electrical pole, with a mighty crash that was heard all over town, causing a blackout until a new pole could be erected.

Down the street was a guy who had converted their lot into a junkyard, where he tried to make a living recycling metals and a few odds and ends. A hard way to make a living; it always amazed me that they had enough to eat. Eventually he gave up and got a job.

Another neighbor accused me of sneaking around their mobile home at night. Well, he had heard something at night, and I was the only guy he ever saw walking around, so it had to be me. He told me that he had taken his gun and shot a bullet right through the thin walls, but didn't hit anything. It was probably an innocent cow, which we occasionally had roaming around at night.

It was almost entirely white people who lived in Dolan, though there was one Native American who lived farther down the hill. He had a Hogan ceremonial hut next to his house, and sometimes I could hear him greet the setting sun with his ceremonial rattles and joyful shouts.

A wild-looking guy lived for a year in a seriously dilapidated hut about 300 yards down the hill. He roamed around on an ancient smoke-belching three-wheeled contraption, with his long hair and long beard flowing behind him.

My neighborhood had other interesting characters. Some drove around with license plates they'd found in order to avoid paying the vehicle tax. There was also a drug house that manufactured methamphetamines.

A poor town does not merit the same services as a more affluent area. That was evident in the mail service. There was only one mail carrier, who had a 200-mile route, so it was really hard to be allowed to put up a mailbox along the paved road. Everybody else was issued a post office box in the little post office in town.

The town had two bi-weekly newsletters for a number of years. They announced the dates for the annual Dolan Days parade and the weekly bingo nights, besides a lot of gossip and some very odd letters to the editor. One newsletter was decently done; the other really needed a spell checker.

We had very good ground water, but it was so deep that few people could afford their own well. Instead, most houses had cisterns and water was trucked in from public wells. The town itself had a small water company, which often had financial problems. Most summers they had trouble meeting the demand of the town, signaling their level of distress with colored flags. Fortunately, everybody had the good sense not to have a lawn in the dry desert. A lesson nearby Las Vegas could learn a lot from.

Despite all the little warts, I liked living in Dolan. Some of the other EIs hated it, but I liked it. The air was clean and the views were fabulous right out the window. The people were friendly. I was often offered a ride when people saw me out hiking around — walking was so unusual that people in my neighborhood called me "the guy who walks."

If my car had had a breakdown, it would surprise me if it took more than five or ten minutes before a friendly guy in a pickup truck would stop and offer help. I once saw a delivery truck break down in my neighborhood and it only took a few minutes before one of my neighbors was on the spot with his tool chest and got the problem taken care of.

There was a barber shop down near the highway between Kingman and Las Vegas. It was a father-and-son outfit. The son would cheerfully do house calls for people who were disabled and could not come to their place.

He only charged four dollars extra for a house call — he could have doubled his entire price and I would have paid it, but that is not the Dolan way.

The little grocery store in town, called "Double D" for some reason, refrained from using pesticides in their store. Solely because they knew it was harmful to the local EIs. The local bank was also very accommodating, cheerfully so, in fact. Even though they only saw me twice a year, they knew who I was.

The house closest to me was a small one-bedroom mobile home, which sat empty for years. Then a guy moved in and started burning his trash in an old steel trash can — magazines, plastic, etc. He worked all day in Kingman and would always burn his trash after sunset, when the cooling air would roll down the side of the hills and put me directly in the highly toxic plume of smoke. Several times he first got started after I went to bed, and each time I had to immediately go away and walk around the neighborhood for a couple of hours. When I got back, any clothing and bedding that got exposed to the smoke was stinky and had to be washed. I could not live with these burnings, which happened about twice a week.

I fretted about how to get him to stop, without making him angry and then possibly making sure to make my life even more difficult. I had heard enough stories about how vindictive neighbors could be, though they all had happened in the Eastern states.

When I went to talk to him, I immediately offered to pay for the trash service to take care of the problem, but he would not hear of it. Instead, he said he would just dump his trash at his job in Kingman. And he did. There was never again a problem.

Not all neighbors were this good. My next-door neighbor refused to call me when the painter was coming to paint her house and her garage, and the guy across the street declined my offer to buy him a tank of propane if he would stop burning wood in February, when the wind tended to come from his direction, but fortunately those were not major problems to live with.

The people of Dolan Springs might not be very educated or sophisticated, but they were real people. What you saw was what they were, none of the pretensions of so many self-absorbed city people. There wasn't any of the "my car is bigger than yours" or desperate attempts to live beyond their means in order to impress the neighbors.

It was a hot desert climate. The summer basically lasted from May until mid-November. The middle of the year was hot and windless, and we didn't get the summer rains to cool it down, like most of Arizona did. The streets of Dolan were completely quiet on summer afternoons, with not even a bird in sight. Even the rabbits would find a low spot in the shade and flatten themselves out so they looked like they had been run over.

When the sun went down, there would be more activity outside. People would come out and tend their yards or work on their houses. Those building houses did it mostly over the winter. A few did it over the summer, working only at night.

The winters were rather mild, with rare snowfall. In the six winters I spent there, we only had a real lasting snow once. The daytime temperature in January was often in the fifties, while it would plummet down to around freezing every night. In February we tended to get the rain, as a cold drizzle together with cold winds from the north.

A desert is not a dead place. There are many animals, but most hide during the day. I would have scores of quail and rabbits coming through my yard, looking for kitchen scraps and the precious water I provided. A few times coyotes would come to drink at dusk as well, though I could mostly only hear them howl at night.

I never saw a bobcat or a mountain lion, but I knew people who did. There were a lot of scorpions, rattlesnakes, black widow spiders and Wallapai tiger beetles, but it was rare that anyone got stung or bitten. After awhile one got used to them, even when finding them in the house. One EI got bitten by a brown recluse spider that was hiding in his boot. A doctor had to suck out the venom, or he would have lost the toe.

The vegetation was mostly tall yuccas and even taller Joshua Trees that look like something from another planet. There wasn't any traffic, agriculture, industry, pesticides, lawns or mining in the area. The only air pollution was the occasional toxic drift of dryer fumes and some wood smoke in the winter.

We never had a real earthquake, but many small ones that sounded like distant thunder and made the garage door creak.

Since I first went on vacation in Arizona fifteen years earlier, I'd always wanted to live in this beautiful state. It didn't turn out exactly like I had envisioned it, but the beautiful surroundings were a definite plus. I think that appreciating the good things in life helps with the bad. So many people with disability and sickness never come to acceptance of their situation but keep wishing for what can't be and are consumed by anger and depression, making their lives much worse than they need to be.

The EI community consisted of a dozen households when I moved there, and we had about one newcomer moving to the area each year. Most of the EIs were married. In two cases, the spouses lived in separate houses, so the healthy spouse had more room and less living restrictions.

It was a stable community, with a diversity of people, including a college professor, a police officer, a school teacher and a machinist. Some people were reclusive, some were outgoing, a few a bit odd.

The EIs in Dolan were generally more functional than those I met in Dallas. Most of us got somewhat better by simply living in the cleaner air and in a stable living situation, where we did not constantly have to watch what all the neighbors were doing. Here we could gradually get a little better, test our limits, and loosen up a bit on our rigorously restricted lifestyle.

Las Vegas was a ninety-minute drive away, with several large health food stores, and anything else imaginable. To get there, one had to drive across Hoover Dam.

The first time I did, I looked at all the low-hanging power lines and wondered if that would be a problem, but I did fine. The next time I passed over, there was a lot of traffic and I had to stop right between two big transformer stations. That did fry me. For the next two weeks, my low-EMF telephone bothered me, for the very first time since I started using it two years before.

The next time I crossed over, I made sure to do it at a time with low traffic and did just fine. The fourth time, there was little traffic and no stopping, but I still got fried and again had trouble using my telephone for nearly two weeks. It would be over two years until I crossed the dam again. I found other sources for organic produce and once in awhile, other EIs would bring me a few items from Las Vegas. A food co-op in Tucson would once a month send up an 18-wheeler with food stuffs to our buying group, and that took care of most of my needs. Then they began to build a bridge over the Colorado River, which promised to reduce travel time to Las Vegas to one hour. Short enough that it was possible to commute to work there.

People started buying up land around Dolan; land speculators roamed around; the prices doubled. And doubled again. But the bridge got delayed again and again. One delay was caused by a big crane falling into the gorge during a storm. The bridge was intended to be finished in 2006, but as of this writing, it is expected to be done in late 2010.

Some people moved out from Las Vegas before the bridge was done. They expected to only have to live with the long commute for a year or two, and get in before the real estate prices really would take off. A new type of people were slowly trickling in.

One couple of such newcomers flew a flag with the Asian Yin-Yang symbol every day. After doing that for a year, I happened to be walking by while they were doing some yard work. They told me that many people had asked about the flag, but I was the first one who knew what it meant.

Another sign of the new times was when I helped push a woman's car out of a sandy wash (dry creek bed). She had dug herself a nice hole with her spinning wheels, so the body of the car was almost resting on the sand. Her car had Nevada plates on it and her tight and revealing outfit was more suitable for the Las Vegas scene than Dolan Springs, where many women were old and wrinkled from too much sun and too many cigarettes, and none of them wore fancy clothes or makeup.

Dolan Springs was a peaceful place, and after all the upheavals of Dallas, that was exactly what I wanted. There wasn't much of a social life there, but the EI community got together for parties a few times a year.

My first year in Dolan was great. I did well there, and in the spring I drove back to Dallas to visit Dr. Rea and Debby. In the fall I spent a week driving around the gorgeous country in southern Utah.

I was summoned for my first disability re-evaluation. Unfortunately the doctor's office was right next to a power line, and he refused my pleas to see me in the parking lot behind the building. Having to be in there for about an hour and a half messed me up so thoroughly that I slept all night in a tent, feeling as if the ground under me was shaking continuously. Of course, it didn't shake; it was my nervous system that acted up from the excessive exposure. It was no better the next morning, but a healer in Sedona pulled me out of it again the next afternoon. I went to see him a few times afterwards, but there wasn't any more he could do for me.

Trouble started during the second winter in Dolan. I found that I didn't do well inside the house, once I had to close it up for the winter. My head was foggy and hurt all the time, and I had trouble tolerating my foods. In January I put up a cot on the front porch and slept there until I moved away four years later.

Soon after, I also became more electrically sensitive. I could no longer drive my low–EMF car, and the heating system in the house now bothered me, so I had to go for a walk two to four times a day while the house warmed up.

Not being able to drive was a sudden and huge problem. The other EIs rallied to help me out by getting me food and things I needed until I could organize a more permanent solution with a hired shopper and deliveries of food by truck and mail. Only one person refused to help, but the others cheerfully made up for it. I bought a freezer, which was put out in the garage, so I could buy more frozen food at a time. Things got organized, and I didn't go without anything I needed, but I could go no farther than I walked. Trips away from Dolan were months apart, and then only on the back seat of the very few cars I could tolerate.

After being stuck for two years, my situation worsened. One new problem was that I had become sensitive to light, which is common among electrically sensitive people. But it took me another year to figure it out, as my symptoms from light exposures were the same as for other types of EMF exposures—light is a form of EMF, so that is not so surprising. My symptoms also tended to show up hours after I had been out in the sun, which I was every day, making it extra difficult to pinpoint.

I hired someone to take me to Dallas for five weeks, at great cost, but it helped. Within a few months, I could start to drive the car again, though I could only drive it about twenty minutes at a time. With rest stops, I could do about 150 miles on a good long day.

I wasted no further time working on an exit plan. I bought a piece of land near another EI community in northern Arizona and had a house built there.

The house was a success. I finally had a safe and comfortable place to live, after ten years.

Appendix: References for Chapter Twenty-Three: Stress Syndrome

Alvarez, Everett, and Anthony S. Pitch. *Chained Eagle*. New York: Dell, 1989.

Ammassari, Adriana, et al. "Depressive Symptoms, Neurocognitive Impairment, and Adherence to Highly Active Antiretroviral Therapy among HIV-Infected Persons." *Psychosomatics* 45 (5), September–October 2004, pp. 394–402.

Anderson, Terry. *Den of Lions*. New York: Random House, 1993.

Ballweg, Mary Lou. "Psychologizing of Endometriosis." *Clinical Consultations in Obstetrics and Gynecology* 7 (3), September 1995.

Bertschler, John, et al. "Psychological Components of Environmental Illness: Factor Analysis of Changes During Treatment." *Clinical Ecology* 3 (2).

Bing, Eric G., et al. "Psychiatric Disorders and Drug Use Among HIV-Infected Adults in the United States." *Archives of General Psychiatry* 58, August 2001, pp. 721–758.

Black, Donald, et al. "Environmental Illness: A Controlled Study of 26 Subjects with '20th Century Disease.'" *Journal of the American Medical Association* 264 (24), December 26, 1990, pp. 3166–3170.

———. "The Iowa Follow-Up of Chemically Sensitive Persons." *Annals of the New York Academy of Sciences* 938, March 2001, pp. 45–56.

———. "Measures of Distress in 26 'Environmentally Ill.'" *Psychosomatics* 34 (2), March–April 1993, pp. 131–138.

Caress, Stanley M., and Anne C. Steinemann. "A Review of a Two-Phase Population Study of Multiple Chemical Sensitivities." *Environmental Health Perspectives* 111 (12), September 2003, pp. 1490–1497.

Frank, Anne. *Anne Frank: The Diary of a Young Girl*. New York: Washington Square Press, 1972.

Gibson, Pamela Reed, et al. "Chemical Sensitivity/Chemical Injury and Life Disruption." *Women and Therapy* 19 (2), 1996, pp. 63–79.

———. "Disability-Induced Identity Changes in Persons with Multiple Chemical Sensitivity." *Qualitative Health Research* 15 (4), 2005, pp. 502–524.

Hardell, Lennart, et al. "Secret Ties to Industry and Conflicting Interests in Cancer Research." *American Journal of Industrial Medicine* 50 (3), March 2007, pp. 227–233.

Huss, Anke, et al. "Source of Funding and Results of Health Effects of Mobile Phone Use: Systematic Review of Experimental Studies." *Environmental Health Perspectives* 115 (1), January 2007, pp. 1–4.

Kovic, Ron. *Born on the Fourth of July*. New York: Pocket Books, 1977.

Krell, Robert. "Holocaust Survivors: A Clinical Perspective." *Psychiatric Journal, University of Ottowa* 15 (1), November 1990, p. 238.

Kreutzer, Richard, et al. "Prevalence of People Reporting Sensitivities to Chemicals in a Population-Based Survey." *American Journal of Epidemiology* 150 (1), July 1, 1999, pp. 1–12.

Levine, M. "Listening for 18 Seconds." *New York Times*, June 1, 2004.

Linnell, Dolores, and Simon Easton. "The Relationship between Phobic Travel Anxiety and the Physical Symptoms of Whiplash Injury." *Rehabilitation Psychology* 49 (4), November 2004, pp. 317–320.

McDaniel, Eugene B., Captain, U.S. Navy, with James Johnson. *Scars and Stripes.* Irvine, CA: Harvest House, 1975.

Michaels, David. "Doubt Is Their Product." *Scientific American* 292 (6), June 2005.

Patterson, D., et al. "Post-Traumatic Stress Disorder in Hospitalized Patients with Burn Injuries." *Journal Burn Care Rehabilitation* 11 (3), May–June 1990, pp. 181–184.

Platt, Mary Frances. "The New Refugees." *Ragged Edge*, March–April 2003.

Roca, R., et al. "Post-Traumatic Adaptation and Distress Among Adult Burn Survivors." *American Journal of Psychiatry* 149, September 1992, pp. 1234–1238.

Sickmann, Rocky. *Iranian Hostage: A Personal Diary.* Topeka, KS: Crawford Press, 1982.

Siegel, Bernie, M.D. *Love, Medicine and Miracles.* New York: Harper & Row, 1986.

Siegel, Shepard, and Richard Kreutzer. "Pavlovian Conditioning and Multiple Chemical Sensitivity." *Environmental Health Perspectives* 105 (Suppl. 2), March 1997, pp. 521–526.

Sorg, Barbara, and Balakrishna Prasad. "Potential Role of Stress and Sensitization in the Development and Expression of Multiple Chemical Sensitivity." *Environmental Health Perspectives* 105 (Suppl. 2), March 1997, pp. 467–471.

Speed, Nancy, et al. "Post-Traumatic Stress Disorder as a Consequence of the POW Experience." *Journal of Nervous and Mental Disease* 177 (3), 1989, pp. 147–153.

Tyre, Peg. "Battling the Effects of War." *Newsweek*, December 6, 2004.

Watts, David L. "Auto-Immune Disease and Women." *Townsend Letter for Doctors & Patients* 238, May 2003, pp. 64–69.

Zavestoski, Stephen, et al. "Patient Activism and the Struggle for Diagnosis: Gulf War Illnesses and Other Medically Unexplained Physical Symptoms in the U.S." *Social Science and Medicine* 58 (1), January 2004, pp. 161–175.

Bibliography

Aron, Elaine. *The Highly Sensitive Person.* New York: Broadway Books, 1997.
_____. *The Highly Sensitive Person in Love.* New York: Broadway Books, 2001.
Becker, Robert O., M.D. *Cross Currents: The Perils of Electropollution — The Promise of Electromedicine.* New York: Tarcher, 1990.
_____, and Gary Selden. *The Body Electric.* New York: Quill, 1985.
Brennan, Barbara. *Hands of Light.* New York: Bantam, 1988.
Castleman, Barry I. *Asbestos: Medical and Legal Aspects.* 4th ed. Englewood Cliffs, NJ: Aspen Law and Business, 1996.
Granlund-Lind, Rigmor, and John Lind. *Black on White: Voices and Witnesses about Electro-Hypersensitivity: The Swedish Experience.* Sala: Mimers Brunn, 2005.
Klass, Perri. *A Not Entirely Benign Procedure: Four Years as a Medical Student.* New York: Plume, 1994.
Nordstrom, Gunni. *The Invisible Disease.* New Alresford, Hampshire, UK: O Books, 2004.
Randolph, Theron, and Ralph W. Moss. *An Alternative Approach to Allergies.* Rev. ed. New York: Harper & Row, 1989.
Shilts, Randy. *And the Band Played On.* New York: St. Martin's Press, 2000.
Smith, Cyril W., and Simon Best. *Electromagnetic Man.* London: J. M. Dent, 1990.
Zwillinger, Rhonda. *The Dispossessed.* Paulden, AZ: The Dispossessed Outreach Project, 1999.

The many books by Dr. Sherry Rogers, M.D., as well as her newsletter, are all available from prestigepublishing.com.

Index

dehumidifier 61
dentist 9, 57, 85
desert animals 207, 219
desert environment 32, 213
detox cocktail 25, 40
detox procedures 39
diagnostics 7, 9, 23, 24, 26
diesel fumes 6, 60
disability: evaluation 135, 168, 190, 221;
 insurance 134, 138, 139, 140, 150
doctors: orthodox 7, 26, 29, 33, 37, 38,
 177, 189, 191; unhelpful 12, 31, 33, 34, 36,
 37, 84, 138, 168, 172, 173, 175, 189, 191,
 221; visiting 23, 156; see also medical
 clinics
Dolan Springs 207, 213, 215
driver's license 146
driving test (EMF) 72, 88, 108
drugs 32, 144, 161; see also antibiotics
dryer sheets 42; see also laundry products
dust mites 19, 132
dysfunction 119, 151, 153, 158, 159, 171

education 84
EI premium 118
electric fences 82
electrical sensitivity 48, 65, 70, 74
electrical transformesr 85, 96, 220
electromagnetic hypersensitivity 77; car
 72, 77, 86, 88, 90, 128, 160, 199, 202,
 204, 221; reduction 67, 71, 86, 151, 184,
 195; shielding 201; sources 68, 79, 80,
 82, 85, 121; symptoms 9, 54, 65, 68, 70,
 72, 75, 80, 88, 90, 103, 114, 137, 148, 149,
 156, 165, 195, 199, 201, 208, 220, 221;
 travel 80, 162; see also driving test
 (EMF); gaussmeter; powerline
emotional impact 167
emotional responses 67, 71, 73, 107, 171,
 219
energy accumulation 105
energy healing 73, 80, 85, 105, 155, 221
Environmental Health Center 22, 39, 123
 190
extreme situations 170
Exxon Valdez 123
eye symptoms 31, 33, 55, 82, 106, 152

fabric softeners 15, 42, 60, 62, 156
family support 113, 132, 136, 150, 210
fatigue 55
fax machines 121
flame retardants 35, 36, 56, 70
floor 61; see also carpet; tile floor
food 18, 19, 23, 57, 158; allergies 7, 9, 19,
 29, 63, 129, 158, 187; chemicals 19;
 organic 19, 100; rotation 8, 41, 60
formaldehyde 60, 84, 180, 190

fragrance policy 38, 126
fragrances 15, 20, 26, 27, 38, 54, 56, 57,
 123, 168
fragrant patients 26, 27, 38, 126
frequencies 197
fried dust 204
furniture 21, 49, 98

gas heat 62, 212
gasoline 5, 17, 18
gaussmeter 48, 78, 91, 199, 200, 206
glass pots 127
grass, symptoms 32
ground currents 178, 206
grounding exercise 69, 70, 74, 90, 91, 99,
 105, 182
groups see patient groups

hair analysis 24
haircuts 20
health insurance 50, 112, 121, 136, 159, 174,
 197
heart chakra 107
heat 130, 132, 145, 152, 184
helpers 68, 72, 76, 77, 80, 81, 87, 89, 91,
 120, 134, 214, 221
hermits 145
hiking 32, 54, 55, 60
home health care 101
homelessness 76, 103, 140, 142, 147, 149,
 151, 211
homeopathy 37
hotels 32, 33, 34, 166
house hunting 61, 62, 205
human battery 105
humor 41, 99, 143, 196
hyperacusis see sound sensitivity

immune system 25, 26
indoor air quality 12, 14
industry cover-up 10, 172; see also corporate power
ink sensitivity 27, 42, 55, 59, 131, 132, 154,
 188
insect bites 116
insecticides 11, 32
insulation 185
intravenous feeding 103, 159
intravenous supplements 25, 112

job description 13, 15, 44, 53, 58, 65
job struggle 15, 59, 168, 186

kinesiology see muscle testing

lab tests 9, 24, 40, 134, 164, 190
Lattieri, Dr. Mike 96, 206
laundromat 43, 62